MONKEYS IN THE MIDDLE

Monkeys in the Middle

How one drug company kept a Parkinson's disease breakthrough out of reach

Nick Nelson

For more information about the GDNF trials, including before-and-after video footage of the GDNF patients, please visit: www.monkeysinthemiddle.org.

Cover design: Steve Reed
Interior design: Jaye Pratt, Book Works, Inc.

For more information, contact:
BookSurge Publishing
www.booksurge.com
(866) 308-6235
orders@booksurge.com

ISBN: 978-1-4196-9655-6

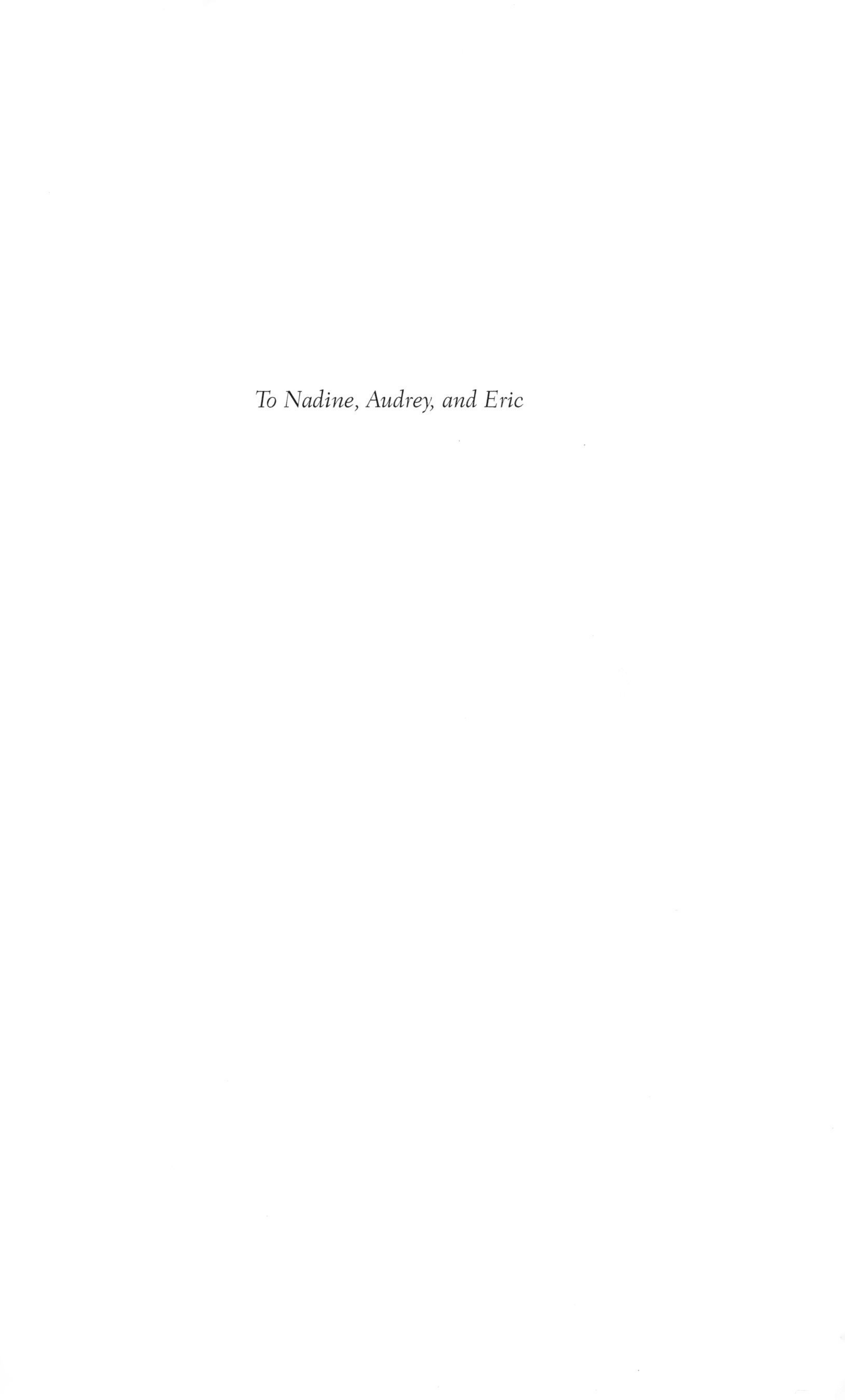

To Nadine, Audrey, and Eric

ACKNOWLEDGMENTS

I would like to give my deepest thanks to the patients, caregivers, and medical experts who assisted me in this work, most of whom are mentioned by name in the following pages. Thanks also to Linda Herman, Paula Wittekind, and those others in the patient community who provided access to people and information and to Loraine De Martino for her editing assistance. Finally, thanks to Paul Osborne for asking me to tell this story.

PREFACE

The writer of the following observations offers them to the public, with the pleasing hope that they may lessen the number of victims to negligence and presumption.

—James Parkinson, "Medical Admonitions," 1799

James Parkinson was a British physician who practiced in Hoxton Square in London. His professional pursuits ranged from politics to paleontology, but his best-known contributions were medical. He published "An Essay on the Shaking Palsy" in 1814 and in it gave the first definitive clinical description of the malady. His success in identifying and describing the disease eventually earned him the dubious honor of having his name attached to it.

Parkinson begins the landmark essay with a disclaimer. He asks the reader to excuse the less-than-scientific means he employs to arrive at his conclusions. Parkinson admits that he had not done rigorous experimentation. Rather, he had observed afflicted Londoners on the city's streets, and he had interviewed them and their doctors in order to better understand the disease. He drew his conclusions from those observations and interviews. Thus, he acknowledges that in the essay "mere conjecture takes the place of experiment" and "analogy is the substitute for anatomical examination, the only sure foundation for pathological knowledge."

I offer a similar disclaimer at the outset of this book. I'm not a scientist, and my research for this book did not entail any experiments (much less anatomical examination). It is true that I have made extensive use of data from medical journals, court records, and other sources, which grounds this account in the "sure foundation" Parkinson describes. The most useful sources for this account, however, have been the patients themselves, as well as their family members and their doctors. I have relied heavily on my interviews with them and on my own observations of the patients with whom I was fortunate to spend some time. The story of the Parkinson's drug "GDNF" is, after all, an intensely personal one.

Parkinson also begs pardon in his essay that the work isn't more complete and refined, and I echo it here. He explains that he feels an urgency to publish because he hopes his description of the disease will accelerate the development of a cure. "[I] therefore considered it a duty," he writes, "to submit [my] opinions to the examination of others, even in their present state of immaturity and imperfection."

INTRODUCTION

Case #1: Stephen Waite

It was a brisk, overcast winter morning in 2001 when Stephen and Margaret Waite drove to downtown Chippenham, a market town between Bristol and Swindon in southwest England. Stephen parked his car in front of the five-story, steel and glass St. Paul office building. He held the front door open for Margaret and they both entered. The couple stood in line for half an hour before a pretty young woman from the Social Security department asked them to follow her to a small, boxy room that was empty except for a desk and three chairs. Most entered that room hoping to plead or cajole their way into new social security benefits. There was a conspicuous red call button on the desk that threatened to bring security guards running if one wouldn't take no for an answer.

The young woman looked bewildered when she heard Stephen's request. The man had handed her a stack of government disability checks, payment slips that he could have exchanged for cash. He was returning them, the man explained with an impish grin. He didn't need them anymore.

The woman looked down at the checks as if unsure what to do. This was highly irregular, she said to Stephen. Never in her experience at the Social Security department had a recipient of disability checks attempted to return them.

Stephen explained that Parkinson's disease had once left him unable to work. Ten years ago, the disease had forced him to apply for the government benefits. But now, an experimental drug was curing him. He now had plenty of work, and he felt guilty accepting government aid. Perhaps the woman knew something about the irreversible nature of Parkinson's disease because she looked incredulous. "All right," she said, "but if you take a turn for the worse, you come straight back." Stephen thanked her and left the room with the grin still on his face. He had no intention of returning to this place.

Stephen was just 27 years old when a doctor said to him, "Stephen, you have an incurable disease called Parkinson's." He was working as a draftsman and an architect at the time, and he had just started a job near his hometown of Chippenham. He was married with two daughters, a toddler and an infant. (His wife Margaret first saw Stephen in a crowded malt shop when she was 14. Stephen was 17 and looking quite brilliant in a white and navy Sea Cadet uniform. She turned to a friend and whispered, "I think I might marry him." Five years later, she did just that.)

After Stephen was diagnosed, the couple decided not to tell family or friends about the disease because they worried it would jeopardize Stephen's employment. They kept the secret for 20 years. Stephen blamed his erratic movements on back problems, but the cover story grew suspect as his condition worsened. In 1990, when he and several coworkers were laid off, it seemed a fitting time to confirm what most people close to him already had guessed.

Parkinson's had spared him the use of his hands, so he still could take on small drafting projects. But his legs had become wobbly and unreliable. He got around with the aid of a wooden cane, but often it was impossible for him to visit a job site, and his work suffered for it. In 1992, he applied for disability benefits and began collecting the government checks.

By the year 2000, Stephen had lived with Parkinson's for nearly 30 years. He would start his day by heaving himself from his bed to the floor, where he would begin an elbow-splitting crawl to the kitchen for his pills. He would swallow 30 of them by the end of the day, but by that time their effect was diminishing. He finally asked his neurologist about brain surgery and was referred to a neurosurgeon in Bristol who happened to be looking for five patients for an experimental drug trial. It is a testament to the misery of late-stage Parkinson's that Stephen didn't balk at what the trial would require. Two pumps, weighing more than one pound each, would be sewn into his abdomen, and thin tubes would connect to the pumps and would be shimmied under his skin from belly to brain. A pair of holes, each the size of a U.S. Nickel, would be drilled into the skull, and a tiny catheter would be passed through the hole, pushed deep into the brain and secured to the skull with screws. He would have to make a monthly trip to the clinic for an emptying and refilling of the pump. This would be done with a large needle through the skin of the stomach. All this for an unproven drug with no guarantees.

At that time, GDNF had been tested in animals repeatedly with dramatic results. In humans the drug had been tested only twice and had failed spectacularly. Patients reported nausea, anorexia, vomiting, weight loss, and abnormal sexual behavior and showed no significant improvement in their Parkinson's symptoms. But the surgeon in Bristol had designed a new method of getting the drug into the brain. It was possible this drug could relieve some of Stephen's symptoms. It might even reverse the disease.

It was a pleasant thought, but Steven had no real hope of this. By the time he learned of the trial he had lived longer with the disease than without it and had accepted Parkinson's as his companion until death. By participating in the trial, Stephen was donating his body to science, in a way. If the drug proved safe and he improved, science had taken one step closer to a new treatment or cure. If it failed, science knew to look elsewhere. "You may not believe," he said of his mindset of the time, "that I had gotten in such a state that I was thinking more about other people than I was for myself. If it would not have been successful, I still would have felt good about it."

Stephen and four other men became the first humans to have GDNF pumped into their brains. It was a phase I clinical trial—a safety trial whose main objective was to prove that the treatment was safe. Within three months of the first dose, Stephen was more mobile and had better balance than he had had in years. "I could walk from the bedroom to the kitchen. . . . It was amazing—for years I had been falling out of bed and crawling to the kitchen. It was almost immediate, and it was improving."

If GDNF had simply slowed the march of the disease, it would have been a breakthrough. No current drug used to treat Parkinson's could do that much. But the patients reported and the clinical data confirmed that the downhill slide had not only halted, but it had been reversed. After one year the patients showed an average *improvement* of 39 percent on the Unified Parkinson's Disease Rating Scale, the gold standard for gauging the severity of Parkinson's symptoms.

The improvements rippled through Stephen's life in dramatic ways. By the end of the first year, he had stopped using the cane, had cancelled the disability benefits, and had bought a Jaguar XJ-6.

He could drive alone. He could go to the store and shop for trousers, trying them on in the fitting room before buying them, rather than buying them first and trying them on at home, as before. After one year, his other medication had been cut in half. The improvements continued into a second and third year.[1]

At that time Stephen knew little about Amgen, the company in California that owned the rights to GDNF. Amgen had provided the drug for the Bristol trial but had little involvement otherwise and almost no interaction with the patients. In June of 2004, however, Amgen called on Stephen and asked him to share his experience with a roomful of drug developers at a conference on GDNF at the Marriott Grand Hotel Flora in Rome. Amgen was preparing a strategy for bringing GDNF to market, and the purpose of the meeting in Rome was to bring Amgen employees and partners together to discuss how GDNF should be launched globally.

Reading from prepared remarks, Stephen told the group, "Three years on from the surgery there have been rough periods but they are insignificant when compared with the ways I have improved. I can work at my drawing board at any time . . . I also take very little in the way of accompanying drugs, compared to the vast amounts I used before. . . . Life is good and I feel very special to be part of this research."

Stephen returned from the conference and resumed his busy life. His drafting business was thriving, and he was barely keeping up with demand. Parkinson's was still a part of his life, but the disease had retreated enough for him to have a life again. Each month, he would go to Frenchay Hospital to have his pumps refilled. After three years, it had become part of his routine.

Three months after Amgen's conference in Rome, Stephen went as usual to Frenchay for a refilling. But on that day, in early September of 2004, a nurse told Stephen he would not receive any more GDNF. Amgen was halting the trials immediately out of safety concerns. He would need to have his pumps switched off and removed.

Stephen said he would sign anything, he would assume whatever risk, if Amgen would allow him to continue on the drug. He learned that nearly 50 other patients had been receiving GDNF before it was taken away and that many of the patients, like him, were desperate to recover it. When Amgen refused, some of the American patients sued the company in federal court and demanded access to the drug. The process was slow, and Stephen did not know what came of the lawsuit. One year passed and then 18 months.

I met Stephen in late July of 2006, nearly two years after he lost GDNF. He had asked that we meet at a pub near Chippenham because he had moved recently into a smaller home and boxes were piled everywhere. Stephen and Margaret arrived in a small van—they had sold the Jaguar—and when he climbed out, Stephen walked with a wooden cane. He wore a green and white checkered shirt and gray slacks. Margaret walked beside him with a steadying hand on his arm. We sat at a wooden picnic table on the pub's hedge-rimmed lawn under a sagging green and red umbrella.

Stephen is about five-foot-ten, has a stocky build, a ruddy complexion, squinting eyes, and a wry sense of humor. He talks in a sing-song way with the rich, Welsh-tinged accent of the region. He told me that the relapse had not been immediate, as he had feared it would be. There was no abrupt onset of symptoms in the days and weeks after GDNF was withdrawn. Parkinson's crept back into his life in undetectable ways. The symptoms reemerged more gradually than they had disappeared during the trial. Yet certain milestones marked his descent.

The cane was one. He had started using it on bad days a year or so after the trials ended. Now it went with him everywhere, as before. The disability benefits were another. A few months before I met him, Stephen had reapplied for the checks he had triumphantly returned three years earlier. Selling the car, selling the house—these were other indicators.

Stephen seemed to be a naturally cheerful person, much more at ease cracking a salty joke than griping about his declining health. He looked uncomfortable with the somber subject of our conversation and attempted often to steer it toward lighter topics. After circling for a while, he finally spoke of losing the drug.

"Having had the illness for so long—for 30-odd years—when they gave me the GDNF, I relaxed too much, possibly. When they took it away from me I had no fight in me anymore. I was close to a nervous breakdown. I was in an awful state. Fortunately, I think now I'm putting myself together." He seemed to answer my other questions cautiously, and he chose his words deliberately as if tiptoeing around deep wells of emotion.

At the end of that first interview, he uttered a sentence that reflected the sad simplicity with which he regarded the past five years. Far away in America, scientists had debated the ethics of Amgen's decision, lawyers had challenged its legality in federal court and patients had condemned it in the press as unconscionable. Removed as he was from these conversations, Stephen did not know what forces took GDNF away from him or what kept it out of his reach. He knew that he once had it, and that it was wonderful, and that it was gone.

"Amgen took away my Parkinson's," he said. "And then they gave it back to me."

1 Parkinson's Disease

The unhappy sufferer has considered it an evil, from the domination of which he had no prospect of escape.

—James Parkinson, "An Essay on the Shaking Palsy"

Parkinson's disease has no cure. When it seizes you, as it has Stephen Waite and some 3 million people worldwide, it doesn't let go. It usually begins with a twitching pinky or a sluggish left foot, but it becomes a slow crush that can last decades—a gradual, irreversible slide toward bodily tremors, muscular rigidity or abrupt freezing of the limbs. The cause of Parkinson's is unknown. Scientists know what it does to the brain, and they recognize its symptoms as it overtakes the body, but no one knows what triggers it. It is generally accepted that Parkinson's results from a combination of environmental and genetic factors. It has been said that genetics cocks the gun, and environment pulls the trigger.

What the disease does to a person is much better understood than how it begins. It attacks the neurons in the brain that produce a chemical called dopamine, a neurotransmitter that the body uses to translate thought into muscle movement. When the brain sends the impulses to muscles to initiate a walk or a run, dopamine helps transmit the message between nerve endings in the brain. When dopamine levels drop, the signal stalls in the brain, and the intent to walk or run remains just that. The muscles never get the message.

Not only are the intended signals stalled mid-transit, but a host of unintended signals dart through the central nervous system when dopamine levels fall. The body loses its ability to "idle" properly, and the limbs tremble and shake even when a person isn't using them. The muscles also may tighten and remain flexed for hours. The pain from these bouts of rigidity can be excruciating.

Parkinson's isn't usually considered a terminal illness because, unlike cancer or pneumonia, the disease itself isn't usually fatal. It kills you indirectly. A Parkinson's patient with impaired balance might suffer a fatal fall, or a patient who has difficulty swallowing may die of aspiration pneumonia. Parkinson's disease may appear on the death certificate, but it usually appears as a secondary or "indirect" cause of death.

It is, nevertheless, a prolific killer. More of a killer, it turns out, than actual killers. In 2004, the most recent year for which such data is available, Parkinson's beat out homicide as a leading cause of death in the United States. The same was true in 2003, when 81 people were poisoned, 670 were suffocated, 2,049 were stabbed and 11,920 were shot. In total, homicide accounted for more than 17,700 deaths in the United States that year. Parkinson's-related deaths in both 2003 and 2004 claimed about 18,000, as reported on death certificates nationwide.[2]

These facts are not pleasant, and one doesn't hear them often in the patient community, where the prevailing tone, appropriately, is one of hope. They are worth considering, though, because unless a person has the disease or knows a patient intimately, he or she will probably never witness the most severe effects of Parkinson's. The average person sets eyes on a Parkinson's patient only when the patient is at his or her best: the medication is working, the limbs are cooperating and the patient feels confident enough to venture out. For reasons of dignity or propriety, practicality or pride, the patient conceals the disease's most hideous face.

The good news is that current treatments can keep that face from appearing often. The mainstay of Parkinson's treatment today is a drug called Levadopa, or just L-dopa. It relieves the symptoms by artificially replacing the dopamine that patients lack. Once ingested, L-dopa travels through the blood stream and is converted into dopamine as it enters the brain. Its effects can be quick and dramatic. It is the miracle drug on display in Oliver Sacks's book *Awakenings* and in the film adaptation. In the book Sacks describes a remarkable summer in 1969 when he gave L-dopa to dozens of patients at a mental institution in a New York City suburb. The patients suffered from the so-called "sleeping sickness" that swept the globe after World War I. They would remain frozen and mute for decades and were thought to be close to brain dead. The disease wasn't technically Parkinson's, but its root cause was a similar lack of dopamine, so Sacks decided to treat the patients with L-dopa. Once he worked out the right dosage, the results were stark. Patients leapt back into life. Men and women who had been like statues broke out with vibrant personalities. Some had not registered the passage of time and were shocked at the aged face staring at them in the mirror.[3]

In the film, Robert De Niro famously plays Leonard, a patient who makes what seems to be a dramatic and full recovery on L-dopa. He catches the eye of a pretty female hospital volunteer. His condition is so improved that the young woman mistakes him for a visitor and is surprised to learn that he is a patient there. They flirt, they go on walks, they dance. The drug's effect wanes as the weeks pass, though, and eventually we see Leonard once again immobile, incapacitated, and ultimately alone in his bed. The situation is less bleak for Parkinson's patients. L-dopa's effects can be significant, and they can last for more than a decade. But the fictionalized scene does highlight the very real shortcomings of the drug. As the years pass, a patient needs ever higher doses to achieve the same effect. A patient will swing between "on" times, when the drug is working and the patient is high-functioning, and "off" times, when the effects of one dose have worn off and the effects of the next have not yet kicked in. The patient's "on" times gradually shorten, and the "off" times lengthen. Eventually, no amount of L-dopa will subdue the symptoms. Like Stephen Waite, a patient at this point will often consider surgery.

Every Parkinson's drug on the market today has this in common: all of them fail to slow the progression of the disease. Today's treatments can keep the symptoms at bay, and they give patients a quality of life unimagined 50 years ago. But Parkinson's marches on. The drugs eventually lose their potency, and the patient is left at the mercy of a merciless disease.

2 Drug Trials, Errors

Just as patients need drugs, drug companies need patients, not just to buy the drugs but also to help to develop them. And in developed countries like Canada, England, and the United States, new treatments must pass through several phases of testing before they can be sold commercially. Generally, drugs are tested first on cultured cells that have been grown in a lab in a controlled environment. The next step is animal testing, typically in mice or rats, then on to more complex mammals like monkeys. If the drug shows promise, and if its negative side effects aren't too severe, it might advance to clinical trials. A clinical trial is a human trial, and it is the gate through which drugs must pass to reach the commercial market.

Each year in the United States, between 3 and 5 million Americans participate in clinical trials, according to the clinical trial tracking group Centerwatch. At any given time, there are between 50,000 and 60,000 clinical trials underway. The most basic of these are called phase I trials or "safety" trials because their primary purpose is to determine whether a given drug is safe—whether there are any harmful side effects. Like the trial Stephen Waite joined in Bristol, these typically include a relatively small number of patients, and usually the patient knows he or she is getting the treatment versus a placebo.

If a drug fares well in phase I, it may advance to phase II trials. These are designed to test for efficacy, to determine whether the drug is any more effective than a placebo. They typically involve more patients than do phase I trials (from a few dozen to several hundred) and include a control group that receives a placebo.

If the drug has been shown to be safe in a phase I trial and effective in a phase II trial, it may advance to a phase III trial. Phase III trials usually involve hundreds if not thousands of patients at multiple locations around the world. Of the three trial phases they are the most costly for a drug company to sponsor and the most definitive in showing whether a drug works. In the United States the Food and Drug Administration must approve new treatments before they can be sold. A company that wants to sell a treatment must make a convincing case for both the safety and efficacy of the treatment.

Drug companies thus rely on patients to bring new drugs to market. Their business model depends on the willingness of volunteers to sign thick documents and submit to unproven treatments. And the patients, for their part, need to get better. Their most obvious incentive to sign the forms and undergo the treatments is the possibility that they might get relief that no drug on the market can give them. A trial volunteer might get a breakthrough treatment three to five years before the patient population at large because of the time it takes for even a safe and effective drug to advance from a phase I trial to the market.

A second incentive, and one that the GDNF patients mentioned often in my interviews with them, is the chance to advance science toward a cure. They know that every cure is preceded by multiple failed attempts, roads that researchers pursue until they dead-end. Given the volume of clinical trials and the relatively small number of true breakthroughs, it is far more likely than not that a clinical trial volunteer will hit one of these dead ends, or at least that they will fall short of their hoped-for breakthrough. Even so, patients like Stephen Waite reason that science will benefit from their participation. Even if the treatment fails, they reason, scientists will have learned what not to do.

However, the possibility exists that science won't learn what it should. For example, scientists might overestimate a drug's potential and continue plodding on through the trees even after the road has dead-ended. In this scenario, which statisticians call type I error or a false positive, a researcher may conclude that a new drug is effective when really the positive results were due to chance or some other unaccounted-for cause. This error can hurt patients by giving them false hope in an ineffective drug. It can also hurt companies, which might spend millions developing a useless drug that it should have abandoned years ago.

Another possibility is that scientists might underestimate a drug's potential. They might conclude that it is unsafe when in fact it is safe or that the treatment is not effective when in fact it is. Statisticians call this type II error or a false negative. A researcher might prematurely declare "dead-end" when in fact the road continues. This error hurts patients in that it deprives them of breakthrough treatments that might have been realized with a bit more effort. One could argue that it also hurts drug companies because the companies miss out on the revenue that the breakthrough treatment would have brought in—like the treasure hunter who quits after digging a 10-foot hole, leaving the treasure undiscovered just a few inches deeper.

3 The Offer

More than one million Parkinson's patients live in the United States, but until early 2006 I had not crossed paths in a meaningful way with a single one of them. There were no grandfathers or grandmothers, aunts or uncles, cousins, friends, co-workers or classmates. I was a business reporter for the *Corpus Christi Caller-Times*, a mid-sized newspaper in south Texas. I covered small business, tourism, port industry, and a lot of Rotary meetings. The paper had two coveted investigative reporting positions, and I hoped to fill one of them after proving myself at the business desk.

In January of 2006, an acquaintance asked if I would be interested in leaving the paper to write a book about GDNF. At the time, I did not know what GDNF was or why those four letters might merit an entire book. The acquaintance was a local physical therapist named Paul who knew I was a reporter. Paul explained that GDNF was a drug that had been used to treat Parkinson's. He said he had a personal connection to this drug. His step-father, Roger, had been one of about 50 GDNF patients who got the drug between 2001 and 2004. Roger was convinced that GDNF was curing him before it was taken away. He insisted that the drug had been reversing his symptoms.

The sponsoring company, Amgen Inc., had halted the trials abruptly in the fall of 2004. The company cited a variety of safety concerns, Paul said, but many in the Parkinson's community suspected it was really just about money. Roger, along with other patients and their doctors, had been fighting to recover the drug ever since. Paul told me that his own mother was Roger's principal caregiver. She would do for Roger the things that the disease kept him from doing for himself. So, like all full-time caregivers, her life was tied up in Roger's condition nearly as much as Roger's. And as Roger had improved on GDNF and then regressed in its absence, her life, too, had been turned upside-down.

Paul asked if I would be willing to research the GDNF trials and write about what I learned. He could pay me roughly what I was making at the paper to work for six months, and he could cover some limited travel expenses. He said he did not expect the book to take sides on the issue, only that it should be thorough and accurate; he would have no involvement in the research or writing of the book. I would have six months to tell the GDNF story and turn in a publishable manuscript. For Paul it was the price of closure.

The story he shared was intriguing, and of course I wanted to help to give this family closure. But I had a small family to provide for, and I was also feeling the tug to settle down, buy a small home and get a good dog. By quitting the paper I would be cutting loose from an established national company and the security and legal protection it provided. I would also be losing health care benefits that I would not be able to afford as a freelance writer. It also was a questionable career move. I felt I was a good candidate for an investigative reporting position at the paper, and marching from the company after only nine months on the job might burn bridges there. I wasn't likely to find a reporting job elsewhere in town, which would mean uprooting to another city for work.

It so happened that an international conference on Parkinson's disease was going to take place within a few weeks of my conversation with Paul, in late February of 2006. The first-ever World Parkinson Congress would bring the Parkinson's research and patient communities to Washington D.C. for a five-day symposium on the disease. Before I turned down the book project, I decided to attend the conference. I wanted to find out how interested the Parkinson's research and patient communities were in getting to the bottom of the GDNF controversy. The trip would also be my crash course in Parkinson's. I knew very little about it at the time, and I had never known personally anyone who had the disease. I had read *Awakenings* and knew of several famous Parkinson's sufferers, but my direct involvement with the disease had been zero. That was about to change.

4 Janet Reno and the Disease-Modifying Drug

I flew to Washington several days early so I could attend the annual forum for the Parkinson's Action Network. PAN was a 15-year-old grassroots lobbying group with several thousand volunteers nationwide. I would attend the PAN forum on Monday and the World Parkinson Congress later in the week.

The forum took place on the first floor of the Holiday Inn on the Hill, which sits on New Jersey Avenue two blocks from the Capitol. It was a cold, clear President's Day, and the federal holiday had the streets strangely empty as I walked from Union Station to the lobby entrance. I bought two yellow legal pads at the hotel gift shop and got directions to the forum. A panel discussion had already begun when I took my seat at one of the 20 or so round plastic tables that polka-dotted the meeting hall where about 75 people were seated. According to the agenda the panel's topic was embryonic stem cell research. After two days of similar panel discussions and briefings at the hotel, PAN would provide a shuttle service to the Capitol, where members would apply their newly honed lobbying savvy to solicit help from members of congress or their staffers.

A wooden podium was at the front of the room, and on either side were tables covered with royal blue tablecloths. The panelists seated at the tables were discussing advances in stem cell research and taking intermittent jabs at President George W. Bush for his stance on its funding—a not-uncommon occurrence in the Parkinson's patient community, I discovered.

We were all seated, but the room teemed with movement. Heads nodded and shook all around me. Elbows pumped, knees bounced, and arms flared out at random. From the left came a steady thump-thump-thump as a man's foot stubbornly kicked the leg of his chair. It was my first time in a room of Parkinson's patients.

A pen and pad of paper lay on the table in front of me, and emblazoned upon each was a drug company logo. I looked around I noticed more logos—on tote bags and flyers and banners. I flipped to the "Sponsors" section of the week's agenda. Of the 12 sponsors listed, 10 were drug companies. Amgen Inc. topped the alphabetical list. At that point I knew little about what I came to understand is a symbiotic relationship among drug companies and non-profit groups like PAN, who need the sponsorship in order to exist. (In her opening remarks, PAN Executive Director Amy Comstock thanked "Amgen, Boston Life Sciences, Schwartz Pharma, [Department of Defense], Novartis, Medtronic and BIO and others" for their sponsorship of the forum. "It takes a lot of money to put on the forum, and we are grateful to the sponsors," she said.) Amgen had donated $50,000 for the 2006 forum and had done the same in each of the two previous years.

The stem cell research panel discussion ended, and a second group of panelists took to the stage and began talking about the regulatory issues that affect Parkinson's research. The panel's moderator was a tall, bearded man named Peter Lansbury, a Harvard

Medical School professor and researcher at the Center for Neurologic Diseases at Brigham and Women's Hospital in Boston. For most in the room, his presentation was probably a review. For me, it was revelatory.

"Parkinson's disease moves very slowly—it does not rear its head until rather late in the disease process," he said. Parkinson's symptoms generally don't emerge, he said, until 70 to 80 percent of the brain cells that produce dopamine have shriveled or died. Generally, it is only when a patient is this far gone that he or she is diagnosed and treated.

"Your brain has an incredible capacity to recover from that initial loss," he said. "Then, as we know, the disease progresses, and of course the symptomatic medications that are available now do not affect the progression of the disease. For a period of time—that may be five to ten years—symptomatic treatment can be very effective, but after that it's not effective at all. So what I would like to talk about is the possibility of just changing the rate of progression of the disease."

He said that today's Parkinson's patient takes only "symptomatic-masking" drugs, drugs that relieve symptoms and mask the effects of a disease but do nothing to slow its rate of progression. His hope was that given the proper incentive a company could develop a "disease-modifying drug," which would actually slow the disease's progression, or even stop it. Such a drug could make conventional treatments like L-dopa last far longer than they do now. More importantly, if Parkinson's were detected early enough and, if the disease were slowed in its infancy, the symptoms of Parkinson's may never emerge during the patient's lifetime. It would be as if the person never had the disease because the patient would never lose enough brain cells for the symptoms to manifest themselves. It might not be a cure technically, but it would amount to one in a practical sense.

"The first drug of that type would be an absolute blockbuster," he said. "Every major pharmaceutical company in the world would love to have that medicine, but the fact is there is very, very little commercial activity in that area."

He explained the paradox by referring to several recent "blockbuster" drugs, those that produce at least $1 billion in revenue in a year. Drug companies have a far greater incentive to tweak or mimic a proven blockbuster like Viagra, which treats erectile dysfunction, than to invest millions in projects that probably won't pay off. The costs of developing a disease-modifying drug for Parkinson's would be enormous because the clinical trials would have to last several years and involve hundreds of patients, he said. Such a drug would also have to be proven safe before it could be brought to market.

"I have to make it safer than Vioxx and I have to run the most expensive clinical trials in history just to find out if it's working," he said. "Those two things combined create a situation where people just are unwilling to take a leap."

As he spoke, a tall woman wearing a mauve and black checkered dress suit entered the room and sank into the seat next to mine. I glanced over and saw a woman with short brown hair, thick glasses and an oddly familiar face. It was Janet Reno, the former U.S. Attorney General.

She had been diagnosed with Parkinson's in the fall of 1995 and announced the news at a press conference shortly thereafter. She was the forum's keynote speaker. I eventually came to understand that she is one of a handful of high-profile patients who command immense respect in the Parkinson's community. When they walk into a room, the collective awe is nearly palpable. Such was the case when Ms. Reno sat beside me. The whispers of her arrival spread in a wave through the audience. Shaking heads craned to glimpse the woman.

Ms. Reno looked directly ahead at Dr. Lansbury, who spoke in closing about the Orphan Drug Act. The impetus behind the act, which became law in 1983, is that drug companies have a natural incentive to develop treatments for the most common illnesses. More patients mean more customers. The result is an overabundance of drugs for common afflictions like pain, inflammation, obesity and so on. Meanwhile, treatments for less-common ailments fall by the wayside. The law gives tax deductions and an extended (up to 20-year) monopoly to a company that will develop a treatment for illnesses that affect fewer than 200,000 people in the United States. It has been a godsend for sufferers of cystic fibrosis, glioma, and for snake bite victims, all of whom make up relatively small patient populations. Because more than a million Americans suffer from Parkinson's, however, the disease doesn't qualify as an "orphan," and the Orphan Drug Act provides no financial incentive for Parkinson's research.

Parkinson's finds itself in a very unenviable position, Dr. Lansbury said, where companies are scared off by the enormous cost of developing useful drugs and have no dangling carrot from the federal government to do so. The result is that Parkinson's patients continue to rely on L-dopa, and America sees more drugs like Nexium. The heavily promoted "Purple Pill" heartburn medicine was developed by London-based AstraZeneca. The company launched Nexium in 2001—at about the same time the patent for its blockbuster heartburn drug Prilosec was set to expire.

"Nexium is essentially identical to Prilosec in every way, yet it became a patented prescription medication that generates billions of dollars a year for AstraZeneca. So as long as [drug companies] can do that, I think that all the carrots in the world are not going to lead them to try to really develop useful medicines."

Dr. Lansbury concluded and the panel discussion continued, but I dwelt on his remarks about slowing the progression of Parkinson's. Suppose a patient was diagnosed with Parkinson's when only 20 percent of the dopamine cells were gone instead of the usual 70 to 80 percent, and suppose a drug was capable of slowing the rate of the disease significantly. It is possible that the patient could live a long, normal life, free from the symptoms of Parkinson's. The disease would war inside the patient's brain, but it would never progress to a point at which the symptoms of Parkinson's would manifest themselves. If GDNF were such a drug, as patients and doctors suggested it was, then it would be by far the most significant advance in the treatment of Parkinson's since the advent of L-dopa in the 1960s. Why, then, would Amgen not bring it to market as quickly as possible? Why would the company keep it on the shelf?

After the panel discussion ended, Ms. Reno rose and approached the podium with measured strides. She spoke slowly and deliberately, slurring words sometimes. The keynote speech was mostly autobiographical, and clearly it was calculated to inspire. She told of taking up kayaking on the Hudson River shortly after being diagnosed, of wading through the Whitewater and Monica Lewinsky scandals and of running for governor of Florida in 2002 after leaving Washington. She mentioned her famous appearance on NBC's *Saturday Night Live* after so many years of being depicted on the program by comedian Will Farrell.

"If you would have told me when I went to Washington that I would be coming through a Styrofoam wall on *Saturday Night Live*,' I would have said, 'You're crazy.' But it was a wonderful opportunity to realize that it is so important that America laugh at itself more often and that America laugh together."

The speech seemed to hit its target. The audience gave a warm standing ovation. Having put politics behind her, Janet Reno seemed to have accepted a new role in the Parkinson's community. She was a matriarch and a nurturer. She couldn't offer a cure, only the assurance that life could go on until such a miracle came along.

5 The World Parkinson Congress

February 22–26, 2006, Washington D.C.

The dark room exploded into applause when he stepped to the illuminated podium. Before him sat two thousand scientists, patients and caregivers who had converged on the capitol for the first-ever World's Parkinson's Congress. Renowned neurologist Stanley Fahn had enthusiastically delivered the man's introduction, but in this room it was utterly unnecessary. In this room, before this crowd, Michael J. Fox was a rock star.

Fox was diagnosed with young-onset Parkinson's Disease in 1991 at age 30 but kept it a secret for seven years. In 1998, he went public with the news and committed to campaign for a cure. He made good on the promise the following year when he testified before a senate hearing on Parkinson's treatment and research. On that day, in the fall of 1999, Republican Senator Arlen Specter introduced him with the observation that "when someone like Michael J. Fox steps forward, it very heavily personalizes the problem, focuses a lot of public attention on it."

He started the Michael J. Fox Foundation for Parkinson's Research a year later; and with his name recognition, his youthful image and proactive approach to chasing down a cure, the upstart foundation quickly swelled to dominance. With direct contributions totaling $29.3 million in 2005, the five-year-old Fox Foundation took in more than the established National Parkinson's Foundation, Parkinson's Disease Foundation and American Parkinson's Disease Association combined.[4]

To many of the patients I met, he is like a patron saint—an intermediary between them and the powers in Washington that give research dollars and take them away. These patients refer to him simply as "Michael" and talk about his activities as if he were an intimate friend. Under the lights, he shifted in his gray shirt and black suit as the applause continued. He was rocking involuntarily to the disease's silent rhythm. A half dozen television cameras trained on him from a platform at the back of the room, and his image swayed on two enormous screens on either side of the podium. When the applause ended, he spoke.

"Thank you, Dr. Fahn, for that gracious introduction," he began. It was the signature, faintly scratchy voice of Alex P. Keaton and Marty McFly—slower now, slurred a little, but unmistakable. "And thank you for all your hard work in organizing this congress. If you'd go down the street and organize the other congress—that would be great too." There was instant laughter. Mr. Fox's political wrangling over stem cell research funding was well known to this crowd.

When the audience quieted, he continued with a speech that was sprinkled with humor but was at its core a pointed criticism of the sluggish progress toward a cure. Basic research in the lab wasn't translating into practical treatment for patients, despite a recent swell in funding. "I did a search on PubMed, and there were 15,000 citations about Parkinson's over the last seven years," he said. "But

I'm not tying my tie any faster." It was the same criticism I had heard from Peter Lansbury earlier in the week: a growing gap between the lab and the pharmacy.

Many in the crowd were nodding their heads, and I knew of a few in the audience who were listening perhaps more closely than most. A rumor had been circulating at the conference that something big was about to happen. There was talk that the Fox Foundation had been pressing Amgen for more information about the GDNF trials. Another rumor from a reliable source said that Michael would mention the trials in tonight's speech. Was it possible Fox would use his keynote address to announce that Amgen had reconsidered? He seemed to be winding down his speech with no mention yet of Amgen or GDNF.

"Before I go," he said then, "I want to say something about clinical trials. We need to improve the way we design and conduct clinical trials. But more important, we shouldn't let inconclusive outcomes lead to a stalemate, or worse yet, an environment of distrust." Any doubt about what he referred to was cleared up in the following sentence.

"There is so much passion around the recent GDNF trials," he said, then paused—a breathless, lump-in-the-throat moment for a few in the crowd.

"As a patient, I'm with you. But I have no easy answers. Can we trust each other to be objective and pure of motive as we figure this out? In the end, this has to be about the patients. After all, isn't that why we're here?" He encouraged greater cooperation between public and private research, and then he ended his speech to much applause.

I knew that some people present would be disappointed that the speech didn't go further. Steve and Maggie Kaufman, for example, had traveled from Chicago to attend the conference. Steve had received GDNF for nine months before Amgen stopped the trials, and he still carried the pumps in his belly, partly in defiance of Amgen's instructions to have them removed and partly in hopes of getting the drug back. Another woman in the crowd had flown in from Kentucky, where her husband, another GDNF patient, was bedridden. She and the Kaufmans had come to the capital to operate an informational booth about the GDNF trials. I suspected that wherever they were seated in the dimly lit convention hall they weren't satisfied with Fox's remarks on the subject.

I was sitting near the back of the cavernous room. To my immediate left sat Dave Heydrick, a neurologist from Maryland that I had met at the PAN forum earlier in the week. I had bumped into him on the way to the keynote speech, and because he was going to the same place we had taken our seats together. He was tall and lean with short brown hair, a mustache and intense, deep-set eyes. He was unique among his neurologist colleagues because, in addition to treating Parkinson's, he also had the disease. His interest in the conference was both professional and deeply personal.

After the speech and standing ovation that followed, the meeting ended with the performance of an interpretive dance. The voice that introduced the dance said the performer was a professional dancer and choreographer from New York City. The announcer said the dance was inspired by the woman's father, who had Parkinson's. The woman appeared on stage in a sheer white leotard and baggy white pants that fell to her shins. Some sort of thick white strap wrapped loosely around her torso. She appeared to be in her mid-twenties and had blonde, shoulder-length hair.

As it caught the light, her pale figure cut a stark image against the blackness of the auditorium. Then the music started—a disjointed, discordant barrage of sounds, with twanging minor notes from a guitar and the irregular knocking of some percussion instrument. And the dancer started to shift, to twitch, to fling one arm high above her head and to twist the other arm awkwardly behind her back. Her arms became tangled in the loose strap that draped around her. She fell to her knees and then to the floor. She was still tangled in the strap, and her head, feet and hands shuddered.

I did not understand. This dance was intended to represent Parkinson's, and yet none of the patients I encountered during my time in Washington D.C. resembled the young woman who now was writhing on the stage. It seemed to me melodramatic, almost comical. As the minutes passed, the movements became more frenetic until the dance finally ended as it had begun, with the woman standing still and pale white against the black backdrop.

When it was over, I turned to Dave Heydrick for his assessment. I suppose I was expecting a bemused look or maybe a roll of the eyes. But when the lights came on, I saw that his eyes were wet and his face was absolutely serious.

"I never want to get to be like that," he said, still looking at the stage. Clearly, Dave Heydrick had seen something in the woman's dance that I had missed.

6 Before and After

I had come to Washington D.C. to find out whether GDNF was still relevant to the Parkinson's community. The fact that Michael himself had mentioned the trials specifically in his keynote address was perhaps all the evidence I needed. Any doubt that might have remained evaporated two days later, when I saw the before-and-after footage of two of the original Bristol patients.

I first saw the video as it played in a loop on a laptop computer in a noisy exhibition hall of the D.C. convention center. Near the hall's main entrance, dozens of drug company reps stood beside inviting, colorful booths. They were young, attractive and sharply dressed. They handed out pens and pins and little bags of M&Ms with candy shells the same color as a newly launched pill. Farther into the room were the smaller, cheaper booths of the research and patient advocacy groups like the Parkinson's Disease Foundation and the Michael J. Fox Foundation. Behind those booths, a catering crew was serving up assorted hors d'oeuvres, and the room smelled of heavily seasoned meat.

Near the back, in a corner that most people would miss, a group called the Parkinson's Pipeline Project had rented half of a booth space. The Pipeline Project operates a Web site that gives regular updates of promising treatments in development. The Pipeline Project had been following and chronicling the development of GDNF before it was shelved, and then the group had actively pressed Amgen to return the drug to the patients.

A collapsible plastic table filled most of the small booth space, and on top of the table was the laptop. On the screen, a grainy video appeared to be playing in a loop. Any audio on the tape was drowned out by the echoing chatter of the exhibition hall, but the message was clear enough.

In the video, which I was later able to review in some detail, a red box appears on the screen with the words, "Before GDNF treatment: Man with Parkinson's moving hands as quickly as he can. Frenchay Hospital, Bristol."

The box fades and a white-haired man appears sitting at a wooden desk and wearing a black short-sleeved polo shirt. On the desk, about one foot apart, are two black dots the size of pennies. The man moves his right hand back and forth between the two dots laboriously, like a windshield wiper at a very low setting. He then does the same with the left hand. His hand is cupped slightly with the palm down. On his face is a look of intense concentration, and his head follows the movement of his fingers back and forth, back and forth.

The image fades and another red box appears: "After GDNF treatment: The same man moving hands as quickly as he can." Now the man appears wearing a long-sleeved button-down shirt with vertical stripes. His right arm is almost a blur on screen as his hand darts between the two points. His index finger finds the mark, and he maintains the tap-tap-tap-tap-tap at a rate of nearly three taps per second.

The image fades to another red box: "Before GDNF treatment: Walking to the end of the room and back." Now the same man appears in what looks like a makeshift film studio, seated in a wooden chair. The floor in front of him is bare and a white sheet hangs behind him. At some inaudible signal, he pushes down on the arms of the chair to hoist himself to his feet and leans forward so far that he appears ready to topple forward. At the last moment, his left foot juts out and then his right in a disjointed succession of quick stutter-steps that propel him, haltingly, forward. The camera pans slowly to the right and the man's goal comes into view: a black line on the ground perhaps 15 feet from the chair. He moves to circle round the black line and slows, nearly to a stop, as he executes the 180-degree turn. It takes him a full seven seconds to complete the turn, and then he stutter-steps back to the chair, where he sets his left hand on the left armrest, pivots awkwardly, and falls into a sitting position. The entire trip takes about 20 seconds.

Another red box: "After GDNF treatment: Same man walking." This time the red box has barely faded and the man is up, out of the chair and taking swift, steady strides across the room. When he arrives at the black line, he steps easily around it, marches back to the chair and slips easily into it. Round trip in seven seconds.

Later in the video, a second man appears and completes the same tasks. In his case, the walk across the room is so laborious and excruciatingly slow that the pre-GDNF clip is actually truncated, edited for length. In the post-GDNF assessment, he ambles easily across the room and back to the chair in 10 seconds.

I learned that the men were patients from Bristol, England and were among the first few humans to have GDNF pumped into their brains. The trial was small, designed simply to determine whether the drug was safe. The profound results attracted international media attention in 2001 and made the Parkinson's patient community aware of a potential breakthrough in the pipeline.

The video was put together by a British man named Tom Isaacs. Like Stephen Waite and Michael J. Fox, Tom suffered early-onset Parkinson's. He was diagnosed when he was 27. In 2003, he gained some notoriety when he began a 4,500-mile walk around the United Kingdom's coastline that would last one year. The purpose of his epic walk was to raise money for Parkinson's research. Along the way, he visited hospitals and research centers to find out what advances were being made in the treatment of Parkinson's. When his trek took him through Bristol, he met Dr. Gill and the others involved with the GDNF trials. They told him about the drug's history and introduced him to some of the original patients. At the time, the Bristol trial was in full swing. Five patients had been having GDNF pumped into their brains continuously for two years and were showing sustained improvements.

Tom was so impressed with Dr. Gill's trial that he earmarked any money he would raise for GDNF research. He founded a nonprofit group called Movers & Shakers to help fund promising Parkinson's research. Unfortunately for Tom, the GDNF trials were halted before the $700,000 he raised could be dispersed. The money sat, unused, in a bank account while Tom waited for the GDNF trials to get back on track. Tom remained close to the issue and kept in touch with the Bristol patient and doctors.

Tom had made the video in the hope that the Parkinson's research community could not ignore its powerful images. Whatever effect it had on the research community at large, the grainy video would have a career-changing impact on me.

7 Decision

I gave my two-week's notice to the paper on the day I returned from Washington. When the managing editor learned I was leaving, he called me into his office and said that one of the paper's investigative reporter's had accepted a job elsewhere. It had already been decided "at the highest levels" that I was to be her replacement. The new job would mean a 20 percent raise and an extra week of vacation. It would also mean getting away from the grind of story-a-day deadlines and a chance to take on in-depth projects.

It was the job I had hoped for when I joined the paper. It would pay enough to get us into a small house. But after what I had seen in Washington D.C., I couldn't walk away from the GDNF story. I accepted the book deal on the condition that it be stated in my contract that there was no expectation that the book would take sides. With the support of my wife, I left the paper and its many deadlines for a job with just one: I had six months to learn the GDNF story and write it down.

8 Origin of GDNF

GDNF is a clunky acronym for the even less accessible "glial cell-line derived neurotrophic factor." I refer to GDNF as a drug, but it is technically called a biologic because GDNF is produced naturally in the human body. Each of us is born with certain quantities of GDNF in our brain. Scientists don't try to create biologics like they do pharmaceuticals. Rather, they try to re-create what already exists in nature; they develop man-made versions of naturally occurring molecules.

Most brief histories of GDNF begin with a "Eureka!" moment in the laboratory of a small biotechnology company in Colorado. Those histories, however, sever the discovery of GDNF from the chain of breakthroughs that made it possible. A good place to begin may be the birth of Jonas Salk in New York City in 1914. His parents were Russian immigrants, and neither had attended college, but both had high ambitions for their children. Salk, the oldest of three, later said he had no particular affinity for medicine in his youth: "As a child I was not interested in science. I was merely interested in things human, the human side of nature. . . . That's what motivates me. And in a way, it's the human dimension that has intrigued me."[5]

In 1955 Salk became an international hero when he announced that his team at the University of Pittsburgh had developed a working vaccine for polio. When he was asked the same year by CBS journalist Edward R. Murrow on the news program *See It Now* who would own the patent rights to the new vaccine, Salk famously answered, "Well, the people, I would say. There is no patent. Could you patent the sun?" Five years later he founded the Salk Institute for Biological Studies in San Diego on a mesa overlooking the Pacific ocean. His premise for founding the institute, and the mantra of the institute today, was that basic research in biology "is where cures begin."

Dave Schubert, who heads the Cellular Neurobiology Laboratory at the institute, joined the Salk faculty in 1970 after postdoctoral work in Paris. Salk expects most of its faculty to secure both their salary and their research funding through federal grants, overwhelmingly from the National Institutes of Health. For 36 years, federal grants have paid for 100 percent of Schubert's salary and research.

One of his first projects at Salk was an experiment in which he attempted to pull new cell lines from brain tumors in rats. Most cell lines have a limited life span, and they will stop splitting after a finite number of divisions. An established, or "immortalized," cell line, on the other hand, can divide indefinitely, providing a bounty of material for scientists to study. To researchers, they are superior to typical cell lines in the way a freshwater spring is superior to a canteen.

Schubert's team, on the advice of a scientist whom Schubert had met in Paris, injected a toxic chemical into the bodies of pregnant rats. The offspring of those injected rats developed brain tumors; and inside those brain tumors, Schubert found an abundance of mutating, immortalized, cell lines. Schubert published his findings in 1974 in the science journal *Nature* and reported that his team had extracted 120 new cell lines. The article provided a table that described the characteristics of 22 of them. Twelfth on the list is a cell line named "B49." No one knew it at the time, but floating inside the B49 cell line was a potent protein that would one day be isolated and named GDNF.[6]

Consistent with its founder's philanthropic ideals, the Salk Institute made the cell lines available to dozens of research institutions over the years, and scientists worked to unlock their potential. Until the early 1990s, however, B49's went undiscovered. In 1990 Schubert teamed up with a researcher named Martha Bohn from the University of Rochester Medical Center in New York. Bohn recently had published a groundbreaking study that involved mice with Parkinson's-like symptoms. After injecting the mice with a toxin that depleted their natural dopamine levels, Bohn implanted in their brains small bits of tissue from the adrenal glands of other mice. The results were surprising: even though all the tissue died shortly after it was implanted, the effect was a striking recovery in the brain-damaged mice. The parkinsonian mice got better.[7]

Bohn didn't know then (and doesn't know to this day) what exactly in that dying tissue helped the mice improve. However, the study did show that there was some substance that could reverse the effects of a condition very similar to Parkinson's disease. The article fueled a growing interest in finding the growth factor that would protect and perhaps regrow the dopamine-producing brain cells killed off in Parkinson's disease.

Schubert and Bohn decided to search for this elusive growth factor in a few of the cell lines that Schubert had discovered 16 years before. Schubert hand-picked three that he thought were good candidates. Bohn and a post-doctoral student named Jurgen

Engele took Shubert's cell lines, blended up each and splashed the result onto rat cells that had been exposed to toxins. The task was then to determine whether the brain cells bathed in the cell-line soup were more likely to survive than the ones without. It was tedious work. Dr. Bohn later said:

> It would take two or three weeks each time we tested something to get an answer. It was a very long process. You grow the dopamine nerve cells, then you would put medium on from cells we collected from other sources, then grow the cells and see if you get more dopamine nerve cells surviving, which meant counting them all.

The painstaking work paid off. When splashed on the toxin-exposed brain cells, all three of Schubert's cell lines helped the damaged cells to survive. The implications for treating disease were clear: if the cell lines could be used to protect the neurons of someone with a degenerative disease like Parkinson's, it might be possible to actually slow the rate of the disease—something no Parkinson's treatment had ever done.[8]

Bohn's and Engele's work was far from over. They still did not know what in the cell lines had protected the neurons, and until they found it they wouldn't be able to purify it, clone it, and reproduce large enough quantities of it to use as a treatment for neurodegenerative disease. But now they knew where to look. Bohn and Engele found that each cell line had particular strengths, and though all three were promising, the B49 cell line seemed to be the best all around. If a dopamine growth factor were a needle hidden in a field of haystacks, Bohn, Schubert and Engle now knew in which haystack to start searching.

9 Synergen

In 1991, a scientist named Leu-Fen Lin at a small biotechnology firm in Colorado fished GDNF from the B49 cell line after six months of searching. When she and her co-workers realized it was the protein they had been looking for—an undiscovered and, more importantly, unpatented molecule—it was time to celebrate.

"When we finally got the full sequence of the protein, we broke out the champagne," recalled Jack Lile, who was on the team that developed GDNF at Boulder, Colorado-based Synergen. "We knew it was new and novel, and that was a good thing from a company standpoint. Then we realized we can finally patent something."

Synergen was born in 1982 during the so-called "biotech revolution." The revolution began in 1980 with the passage of several key pieces of federal legislation; and most influential was the Bayh-Dole Act, which for the first time allowed universities and other institutions to patent discoveries they made through federally funded research. Prior to the passage of the act, if a study funded by the National Institutes of Health resulted in a new discovery, that discovery simply floated around in the public domain until a private organization snatched it up. With the new law, a university could patent its findings, license its discovery to a private company, and collect royalty checks for the life of the patent.

Synergen was founded by four faculty members from the University of Colorado at Boulder with some venture capital money from a New York firm. Its headquarters on 33rd Street in downtown Boulder was less than two miles from the school's campus; and like a lot of the early biotech firms, Synergen was established as a go-between that shopped the university's discoveries out to deep-pocketed corporations that would market them worldwide. The company eventually developed deep pockets of its own; it grew to 700 employees and built a $75 million research facility in Boulder.

In the late 1980s, its board of directors decided that neuroscience was the most promising niche in the biotech sector, so the company began assembling a team. Synergen hired a neurobiologist named Frank Collins from the University of Utah in 1987 as its first vice president of neuroscience. The company then hired the fastidious Leu-Fen Lin, a specialist in the immensely tedious process of isolating proteins from brain matter and identifying them.

Within two years, Collins and Lin filed their first patent together. It was a protein called ciliary neurotrophic factor or CNTF, and it showed some promise for the treatment of Lou Gehrig's disease, or ALS. (When it was later tested in humans, CNTF caused such significant weight loss that it was temporarily abandoned as a treatment for ALS and explored as a possible treatment for obesity.)

How Synergen's scientists got their hands on the B49 cell line is something of a mystery. David Schubert at the Salk Institute said he has no recollection of having provided it to the company, and the Salk Institute's legal department has no record of a transfer of the material to Synergen. When I contacted Frank Collins at his home in the Seattle area, where he has since retired, he said he could not recall how the company acquired the cell line. He said he believed Leu-Fen Lin had brought it back from an outside lab where she had done some research. "We were never sure where [the B49 samples] came from," he said. "Presumably, Leu-Fen Lin would remember."

When I reached Lin at her workplace at a biotechnology company in upstate New York, she did remember something about the cell lines. She said Synergen already had the cell line when she joined the company in the late 1980s, that it was already sitting in Synergen's liquid nitrogen-cooled tanks when she was hired. She said Frank Collins would know: "If it's anybody, it would be Frank," she said. "He's the cell biologist."

Whatever means Synergen used to acquire it, the B49 cell line became the focus of Lin's attention. After six months of searching, she found the protein she was looking for. Synergen would later name it GDNF. The manmade GDNF was purified and put to the test. Synergen's lab in Boulder doused some extracted rat brain cells with a toxic chemical. Then they smeared GDNF on the same cells and watched to see whether the drug would protect the cells from the toxins.[9]

When the three-week study ended, the effects were obvious—GDNF had singled out and protected the dopamine-producing neurons, the very cells that Parkinson's attacks. Seventy percent of the surroundings cells died, but the dopamine-producing cells remained healthy. In multiple experiments, the cells treated with GDNF survived three times as well as the untreated ones. The scientists also discovered that the cells treated with GDNF grew in size by about a third.

Synergen partnered with Barry Hoffer, a neuropharmacologist at the University of Colorado Medical School, to test GDNF on live rats. The early results looked good: the rats on GDNF maintained dopamine levels far better than the rats without the drug. It was time to let the world know.

The article appeared in the May 21, 1993 edition of the journal *Science;* it described the findings and gave the new molecule a name. The words "glial cell line-derived" refer to the tumor cells from which Leu-Fen Lin pulled the protein. A "neurotrophic factor" is a substance that is secreted by a cell and that helps neurons survive. Once GDNF was proven in rats, Synergen took the next step up the ecological ladder. The company contracted with the University of Kentucky to test GDNF on parkinsonian monkeys. Those tests showed that the protein was equally potent in primates.

GDNF wasn't the only drug in Synergen's pipeline. At the same time it was developing GDNF, Synergen was betting high stakes on a drug called Antril that was being developed to treat septic shock. In the summer of 1994, the FDA declined to approve Antril based on the drug's weak showing in a recent clinical trial. The news devastated Synergen, and the company announced plans to lay off more than half of its employees.[10]

At the same time Synergen was faltering, a 14-year-old company named Amgen Inc. was gaining steam. Like Synergen, Amgen was a young biotech that saw promise in the neuroscience field. Amgen bought Synergen in 1994 for a figure reportedly between $240 million and $265 million. Synergen had other drugs in its portfolio; but, after the loss of Antril, GDNF was the company's star. Amgen's CEO Kevin Sharer later told the *New York Times* that Amgen's scientists had seen before-and-after footage of monkeys treated with GDNF, and the decision to acquire Synergen was an easy one.[11]

"We looked at that movie and said, 'Buy this company,'" he told the *Times*. "Literally."

10 Amgen Early Days

Amgen Inc. was founded in 1980 and, like Synergen, the company cut its teeth on an eclectic mix of projects before settling into human therapeutics. In the early years the company developed organisms that would extract oil from shale and proteins that would make chickens grow faster. Amgen was running out of money in 1983, so it went public and raised $40 million in its initial public offering. The company's first CEO, George Rathman, bet the bank on a breakthrough treatment for anemia, a condition that weakens patients by reducing their red blood cell count. It has now become a part of the corporate lore how 15 Amgen employees holed up in a hotel for 93 straight nights to work on FDA applications for the drug. The FDA, which must approve every new drug sold commercially in the United States, gave the green light in 1989. Epogen became the company's first big seller.[12]

In 1991, Amgen won FDA approval for Neupogen, a protein that boosts white blood cell levels to prevent infection and septic shock in cancer patients weakened by chemotherapy. By 1994, the year Amgen acquired Synergen, Neupogen had worldwide sales of

$829 million and Epogen had sales of $721 million. The two drugs accounted for more than 80 percent of the company's total revenues. Swallowing Synergen was part of an effort to diversify the company's portfolio and to get a foothold in the neuroscience sector.

After acquiring the rights to GDNF in late 1994, Amgen experimented with different ways of getting GDNF into the brain. Because it is a relatively large molecule, GDNF can't reach the brain through the bloodstream. The capillaries that deliver blood to the brain are unusual in that the cells that make up their walls are tightly packed together. This "blood-brain barrier," as it is called, prevents dangerous toxins that somehow get into the blood stream from seeping into the brain. But the barrier also keeps out useful large molecules like GDNF. This means GDNF can't be taken orally or injected intravenously. It will be blocked by the blood-brain barrier.

When Amgen *did* attempt to inject GDNF into the bloodstream of monkeys, the results weren't pretty. "People who were there said it can only be described as explosive diarrhea," said Jack Lile, the Synergen biochemist, who later joined Amgen. Lile said GDNF had apparently caused a severe reaction in the enteric nervous system, the dense mesh of nerves that surrounds the digestive tract. It became obvious that injecting GDNF into the bloodstream was not going to work. It would have to be delivered directly into the brain.

Getting GDNF into the brain of a rat is relatively easy and can be done with a quick squirt from a well-placed needle. To do it in a monkey is more difficult, but a monkey brain is small enough that if the drug gets close to the target area, the GDNF can seep into the parts where it will do the most good. A succession of studies published in the early to mid-1990s showed that GDNF delivered into the fluid-filled ventricles of the brain produced significant results. Other studies showed that GDNF protected motor neurons in the same way it protected dopamine-producing ones, which meant it might be useful for treating ALS and other motor neuron diseases. With each new study, the drug's potential seemed to swell.[13]

Based on the strength of those studies, Amgen decided to test GDNF in one group of Parkinson's patients and one group of ALS patients. The protein would be injected into a ventricle of the brain. The original plan was to enlist 85 advanced-stage Parkinson's patients for a study that would last three years. Between July 1996 and April 1999, 13 women and 37 men underwent surgery. Each was fitted with a thin plastic catheter that plunged, through a hole drilled into the skull, into a ventricle. The scientists knew that if GDNF simply remained in the fluid of the ventricles and the spinal column, it probably wouldn't do much good. Their hope was that the GDNF would migrate to the *putamen* or the *substantia nigra*—two of the structures most affected by Parkinson's disease.[14]

Thirty-eight subjects received GDNF, and twelve were randomly assigned to a placebo group. Instead of getting GDNF, they got an ineffective saline solution. These 12, as it turned out, were the lucky ones.

Amgen ended the studies prematurely because of a host of negative side effects and a lack of improvements in the patients' symptoms. Not only did the surgery itself cause problems, but many of the patients who received GDNF also complained of nausea, vomiting, confusion, delusions, hallucinations, chest pain, and other symptoms. The study authors concluded that GDNF was decidedly potent but not for the better when delivered into the ventricles. They suggested that GDNF might have failed to migrate to the *putamen* and the *substantia nigra,* where the drug might have done the most good. A different delivery method, perhaps one that targeted those structures specifically, might be more effective.[15]

This was the first time Amgen halted clinical trials of GDNF. It happened without much controversy because the benefits of the treatment were dubious, and the negative side effects were legion. The consensus among the scientists involved was that injecting GDNF into the cerebral ventricles had done more harm than good.

At this point, according to several people involved in the GDNF trials, Amgen shelved the drug. The company made GDNF available to outside researchers for animal testing, but no human would get the stuff for another two years. When GDNF did finally make its way into the brain of another human, the results were broadcast around the world.

11 GDNF via Pump

GDNF maintained a devoted following of researchers despites its early failure in clinical trials. A group of scientists from the University of Kentucky had been involved in GDNF testing since the first monkey trials and were longtime believers in the drug's potential, if it could be properly delivered. GDNF was also gaining new converts. One of them was Steven Gill, a consultant neurologist at Frenchay Hospital in Bristol.

Dr. Gill came to Frenchay in 1994 after completing the British equivalent of residency at Hammersmith Hospital in London. As a consultant neurologist he maintains an office at Frenchay and works there several days a week but also has a private practice outside. His clinic at Frenchay is in a narrow, one-story, orange brick building that was thrown up during World War II as a training facility for American medical staff and was later used to treat casualties after D-Day.

Dr. Gill is an inventor. At fifteen he dreamed up a protective, inflatable suit for motorcyclists. A small canister of pressurized air would attach to the suit, and relying on a sort of rip-cord design the suit would instantly inflate if the rider were thrown from the bike. The idea never evolved into a working prototype, but many of his subsequent inventions did. Dr. Gill now has more than 20 patents in the United States and Europe for various surgical devices and techniques.

Dr. Gill gained some notoriety in the mid-1990s when a BBC news crew filmed him doing a trailblazing surgery for the treatment of tremors and Parkinson's Disease. After the footage aired in the United Kingdom and later in the United States, Dr. Gill's private practice flourished. By the late 1990s, Dr. Gill was refining a surgical technique that targeted a minute part of the brain called the *subthalamic nucleus* that is less than one millimeter across. He would use a tiny electrode at the tip of a stiff wire to destroy bits of delinquent brain tissue. Often, the result was an immediate improvement in patients' symptoms of shakiness, rigidity and imbalance.

He found, however, that some patients would improve initially and then relapse into their previous symptoms after several days. It usually meant that some of the deviant tissue had remained, and finishing the job would mean repeating the surgery. So Dr. Gill devised a new system to make those follow-up surgeries easier. He inserted a tiny plastic guide tube into the brain and then fed the wire probe through the tube and destroyed the unwanted tissue. He could then remove the probe but leave the guide tube implanted in case the patient needed an additional surgery later.

About this time, in March of 1999, Dr. Gill first learned about GDNF. He attended a conference in London that was hosted by SPRING, the division of the Parkinson's Disease Society that focuses on developing a cure. He went to a presentation titled "The neurotrophic factors in Parkinson's disease" that was delivered by a Swiss-born neurologist named Franz Hefti, who worked for the drug company Merck. The presentation summarized the many successful animal trials of GDNF and the failed human ones. The gist of it was that GDNF's potential hadn't been realized because the delivery method had been imprecise.

When Dr. Gill saw the presentation on GDNF, he realized that it would be no great stretch to apply his surgical techniques to the delivery of the new protein. In his spare time he began to design a procedure that would use an implantable pump and an ultra-thin catheter to squirt GDNF directly into the *putamen*. The earlier human trials had shown that GDNF doesn't migrate well through brain tissue. In order to saturate as much of the *putamen* as possible, the GDNF would need to be forced out of the catheter under pressure so that it would diffuse as far as possible into the surrounding tissue. If it were simply dripped into the brain, the GDNF might collect in a glob at the catheter tip without absorbing into the tissue.

Dr. Gill's design called for "convection enhanced delivery" of GDNF, which meant the pumps would be programmed to deliver the drug under pressure and drive it out into the tissue. Convection enhanced delivery, however, presented another problem. All the available catheters on the market had, in Dr. Gill's opinion, a common weakness; to understand that weakness, one has to know a little about how a surgeon places a catheter in the human brain.

The catheters used in brain surgery aren't made for burrowing. They are hollow tubes, and their walls are usually made of thin plastic. To insert them deep into the brain, a surgeon follows five steps: First, the surgeon pushes a thin, stiff wire into the brain along the route that the catheter eventually will follow. Second, the surgeon fits a hollow guide over the wire and pushes it into the brain along the length of the wire. Third, the surgeon removes the wire, leaving only the hollow guide tube in place. Fourth, the surgeon inserts the plastic catheter into the guide tube and pushes it down into the target point in the brain. Fifth, the surgeon removes the guide tube, leaving only the plastic catheter in the brain.

The complex procedure allows neurosurgeons to hit very small targets with precision. However, there is a weakness inherent in step five. When the guide tube is removed and the catheter is left behind, a hollow channel remains around the catheter where the guide tube used to be. Suppose that the catheter is .5 mm thick and the guide tube is 1 mm thick. When the guide tube is removed, a channel that is .5 mm thick will be left behind where the brain tissue has been pushed back by the guide tube.

Dr. Gill knew that GDNF delivered under pressure would follow the path of least resistance. If a channel of empty space existed around the catheter, GDNF most likely would reflux up along the catheter track rather than diffuse into the tissue near the catheter tip. The result would be that only limited amounts of GDNF would actually diffuse into the *putamen*. The rest of the drug would flow up along the catheter and attach to tissue that wouldn't benefit from GDNF.

With all this in mind, and with his experience as an inventor, Dr. Gill designed his own catheter. He spent about $80,000 of his own money to have it manufactured and tested. At .6 millimeters, the new catheter was 40 percent smaller than the conventional 1-millimeter catheters in use at the time.

Simultaneously and across the Atlantic, the Kentucky doctors were developing a procedure that also relied on convection enhanced delivery. In late 1999, the Kentucky doctors and Dr. Gill approached Amgen with their new ideas for delivering GDNF. Rather than inject the stuff into the ventricles and hope that the drug reached the target, they would shoot it directly into the putamen. Both groups asked if Amgen would be interested in sponsoring trials. Another neurologist, Michael Hutchinson from New

York University, also had become interested in GDNF and had approached Amgen about doing a similar trial.

Drug companies often sponsor trials that seem likely to bring their drugs closer to market. It can mean an enormous payoff if the trial proves the treatment to be effective. But Amgen, perhaps stung by the two failed trials in the late 1990s, declined to sponsor either one. Dr. Gill and the Kentucky doctors would have to come up with the funding on their own. Amgen did agree, however, to supply the GDNF for free on the condition that Amgen would own the rights to any new discoveries the scientists made during the trials.

Dr. Gill began shopping around for a suitable pump, and the best that he found was at Medtronic, a Minneapolis-based company that specializes in medical devices. The SynchroMed pump is the size and shape of a hockey puck and at just over one pound, it weighs significantly more than one. He asked Medtronic to provide the pumps for the trial for free, but the company declined. Dr. Gill hoped eventually to enlist five patients for the trial, but he had the funds for only one pump, for which he paid about £6,000 ($9,600 U.S.).

Because of Britain's more streamlined (some would say less-stringent) approval process, the Bristol trial started first. The first patient to volunteer was Henry Webb, a retired Welsh miner whose Parkinson's symptoms were prominent on the left side of his body. In Parkinson's, symptoms appear on the side of the body *opposite* to the affected part of the brain, so the pump was to be implanted on the right side of Mr. Webb's brain. Mr. Webb later told a reporter from the *Bristol Evening Post* that he had not deliberated long when deciding whether to enter the trial: "They explained what they would do and I said yes straight away. I thought that nothing could be as bad as what I was experiencing at that time. So they put the thing into me and almost straight away I felt the difference."

Dr. Gill had applied for funding to the Parkinson's Disease Society, Britain's largest and oldest Parkinson's organization. The PDS initially was reluctant to fund the trial, but a few months after Mr. Webb's first dose of GDNF, his improvements already were significant enough to persuade PDS to provide funding for the additional pumps. Between March and September of 2001, four more patients volunteered for the trial. One of them was Stephen Waite, the man who eventually returned his disability benefits to the government. Another was a retired middle school teacher named Richard Hembrough.

12 Case #2: Richard Hembrough

On the afternoon of January 13, 1633, a thunderstorm lashed the village of Keynsham, a small English farming community midway between Bristol and Bath. At about six o'clock that evening, the resolute bell tower of St. John the Baptist Church in Keynsham lurched sideways and collapsed. The integrity of the 360-year-old church and tower had trickled out over the centuries as England's cold rains eroded the lime in the mortar, particle by particle, from between the building's rough-hewn stones.

Rather than resurrect the old tower, the parishioners opted for a new, more stable one at the church's west end. It took more than 20 years, 50 trees and more than 1,000 loads of stone to finish the job.[16] The new tower stands as the village's most prominent feature and marks Keynsham's center.

Richard Hembrough and his wife Patricia live two blocks from St. John's tower in a four-story semi-detached limestone town home. It was built in the mid-1800s on top of an old abbey cemetery. Keynsham's Abbey had been the second largest in England, but a grassy field and a park now stretch where the Abbey once loomed. The Abbey still is literally a part of Keynsham—its stones were used to build homes nearby, including the Hembroughs'.

Richard and Patricia are natives of the Bristol area; they met as teens during a service project for the YMCA. The two were putting up Christmas decorations at Cossham Hospital in another Bristol suburb called Kingswood. Richard was still shy at 18, but he ventured a "Hello" that led to a chat about Richard's scooter, a two-seater.

Patricia, who was 16 and didn't share Richard's timidity, asked for a ride. The couple would later learn that Patrica's grandparents had met while decorating the same hospital ward. The coincidence endowed their budding relationship with a sufficient degree of meant-to-be.

Richard had attended school until age 14 and then had begun a five-year apprenticeship as a carpenter and joiner at W.J. Hembrough and Sons, a construction company his grandfather had founded. He was not coordinated enough for athletics but enjoyed working with his hands. After his apprenticeship, he studied for two years at Bath Technical School while dating Patricia regularly. The two moved to Newcastle to continue their studies, and they decided to move in together. When they returned to Keynsham during winter break, Richard and Patricia announced that they would be married on Christmas day. The preacher was booked, so they settled on December 30.

Patricia became a dentist who specializes in treating children and disabled adults. Richard earned a teaching certification and accepted a job at Hale Middle School in the county of Surrey. By that time the Hembroughs had two children—a boy and a girl—and the couple had two more boys while Richard taught at Hale.

It was while teaching at the middle school that Richard began to feel the burden of Parkinson's: "I taught drama, I taught math,

English, history, science, cooking. And I didn't have a minute to spare. I felt very lethargic and sick. I felt as if I could eat a horse, but as soon as I started eating, it wasn't very good. My legs were aching constantly. I just had no desire to work or do anything. My face, I know, was changing shape."

He attributed all this to the stress of the job. So after 10 years at Hale, Richard quit and returned to Keynsham to work for W.J. Hembrough and Sons. Richard's father had taken over the business and had hoped Richard, his eldest son, might do the same, but Richard preferred being at the job site to sitting in the office, and, in any case, his health was deteriorating quickly.

In 1982, Richard heard a radio program about Parkinson's disease. A Parkinson's patient was interviewed, and as the patient listed 10 common symptoms of the disease. Richard realized he had experienced almost every one. He contacted a neurologist who interviewed Richard and subjected him to several tests. Richard remembers the conversation with his neurologist this way:

"I'll tell you what's wrong with you."

"I think I know."

"Go on then."

"Parkinson's disease."

"Yep, well done."

Richard was 40 years old at the time. To Richard, it all added up—his difficulty at Hale, his recent struggles just getting around, and perhaps even his hampered coordination during his youth. The neurologist prescribed L-dopa, and Richard improved immediately. The L-dopa gave him back his life for almost 10 years. He would still vacillate between "on" and "off" times, but he was "on" almost all of the time. He was productive at work, and when he and Patricia found a beautiful but run-down town home near St. John's church in Keynsham, he felt up to the chore of restoring it.

In the mid-1990s, the disease began to outpace the drug. Richard's "off" times lengthened and his "on" times weren't as good. By the late 1990s, L-dopa was doing little for him. "One minute I could move, and the next I couldn't, even when crossing the road. People didn't understand and thought I was drunk. I had my driving license taken away."

"Unreliable" is how Richard said he felt. He didn't know, in a given moment, whether his body would respond to his wishes in the next. When he walked, he did so in short, jerking stutter-steps, as if his shoelaces were tied together. His face tightened and deadened into the parkinsonian mask, and he lost the senses of taste and smell. The color seemed to be draining from his life, and he drooped into a general melancholy and insouciance. Finally, he asked Dr. Gill, his neurologist at the time, about other options. He didn't like any of them.

Until the late 1990s, the most common surgery was the pallidotomy, where a surgeon would use a tiny electrode on the tip of a stiff wire to burrow into the brain and destroy bits of the *globulus pallidus,* a structure that is overactive in Parkinson's patients. The surgery can relieve tremor and rigidity, but it doesn't slow the advance of the disease.

In 1997, a new procedure called deep brain stimulation, or DBS, emerged. With DBS, a neurostimulator the size of a pocket watch is sewn under the collarbone. A wire is threaded under the skin, through a hole in the skull to a miniscule electrode lodged deep in the brain. Like a pacemaker for the brain, the stimulator fires off tiny shocks that block the haywire impulses that cause tremors and other Parkinson's symptoms. In studies, DBS has proven effective in about two-thirds of patients.[17]

"I didn't want to go through anything that would remove bits of my brain because I felt I needed all of it, and I didn't want Deep Brain Stimulation because I felt that was making me into a robot,"

Richard later said. "But I said, 'Anytime you get something really good in, I'll be prepared to do it.'"

It was almost two years later that Dr. Gill told Richard about an experimental drug called GDNF. The procedure would be every bit as invasive as the others Richard had turned down, but unlike the others, GDNF had the potential to actually slow the disease's rate of progression.

Richard later said it was not a difficult decision: "I thought, if they're going to try something as big as putting a growth factor in my brain, then it must be something that is going to be worthwhile. I just felt confident about that." Richard said he also felt confident in Dr. Gill's abilities as a surgeon. When he asked Patricia what she thought of the GDNF trial, she said she would support him, whatever he decided.

Patricia later said, "I talked to a colleague recently, who said she thought Richard was being very brave to do something like have the pumps inserted and everything. I said, 'Well, he didn't feel he was being brave because, really, there was nowhere else for him to go.' The medication, which over the years had been successful to a point, was becoming less so. The side effects were becoming greater from the medication, and there was nowhere else to go, really."

Richard's surgery in July of 2001 spanned two days. On the first day, Dr. Gill fastened a metal stereotactic frame to Richard's skull with stainless steel screws. Dr. Gill would use the frame to triangulate in Richard's brain the location of the *putamen*. When Richard awoke on the afternoon of the first day, he had a splitting headache and found it difficult to eat and to sleep with the shiny metal frame surrounding his brain, as if holding his head prisoner.

On the second day, Dr. Gill drilled two holes in the top of Richard's skull and threaded the new catheters into Richard's brain. He implanted two pumps—one on either side of Richard's abdomen—and connected the pumps to the catheters with a tube that he shimmied under the skin of Richard's chest and neck. Richard became the fourth patient to receive GDNF, following Henry Webb, Stephen Waite and another man at Frenchay. A fifth patient followed Richard by a few weeks, and the study was underway.

Richard went home two days after the surgery, but he was back at Frenchay within two weeks. A painful pocket of fluid had formed on his neck, and Dr. Gill's assessment was that some germ had entered Richard's body along with the hardware. He decided to remove it all—the pumps, catheters and tubes—and replaced it with new equipment. About a month after his first surgery, Richard went under the knife a second time. Dr. Gill cut along the same scars to reinsert the pumps. It wasn't until he had returned home from the second surgery that Richard began to see the effects of GDNF.

Course on GDNF

Richard was 56 years old when he began on GDNF. He had been diagnosed at 40 and had lived with Parkinson's for almost 27 years. Before he began the trials, his motor score on the Unified Parkinson's Disease Rating Scale (UPDRS) was just under 40. The other patients' scores ranged from 25 to 42; a healthy person will have a score of zero.[18]

After six months on the GDNF, Richard's motor score had dropped to less than 25, and that was when he was assessed without any medication other than GDNF. When he took a small dose of L-dopa, his motor score fell to less than 10. He had regained his ability to taste and smell and his sexual function was revived. After two years on GDNF, Richard's off-medication score had dropped to just above 15 and his on-medication score hovered near 5.[19]

At first Richard found it rather difficult to gauge his improvements. He had begun to suffer from severe lower back pain that eventually was traced to a congenital defect. Dr. Gill performed three surgeries to correct the defect, and it wasn't until the third was complete—nearly a full year after he began on GDNF—that Richard really could appreciate what GDNF was doing for him.

He described the sensation as a gradual "building up" of stability, strength and confidence. The changes from one day to the next were not dramatic, but the cumulative change was. Every so often Richard would realize just how far he had come:

"I stood up one day, and as I stood up straight I could feel my legs and my body and arms suddenly becoming very stable, strong and stable. That was one of the best experiences. It was fantastic."

Richard said that before GDNF he worried about going to sleep because he would sometimes wake up with his face buried in a pillow and would be powerless to move. While on GDNF he could turn easily in bed, and he could sleep better because his muscles didn't ache as they did before. His hearing and his speech improved, and his "off" time dwindled. "Eventually I had no 'off' time. I didn't go 'off.' I just stayed 'on,'" he said.

During the trial, each of the five Bristol patients also took a drug called Sinemet, an L-dopa-based compound sold by Merck. After about a year on GDNF Richard had stopped taking the Sinemet and the other supplemental medication, he said, because he knew he didn't need them anymore. At first he would skip the occasional dose because he would simply forget. When he found that his "on" time persisted even without the Sinemet, he skipped doses more frequently. Eventually he stopped taking the drugs altogether. He applied for and received a new driver's license and began to venture out around town. "I got more confident, he said. I could go out and do things without looking like some drunken something."

Richard has a good friend named Bob Isaacs, an interesting fellow who shuns motorized transportation and makes a living doing field research for American author Stephen King and others. He is tall, tan, and lanky with long gray hair which he usually pulls back into a ponytail. Bob has known Stephen's family for 25 years, since he was laid off from a job and began washing windows to make ends meet. He knocked on the door of Richard's mother, who gave him some work. He eventually began doing odd jobs for Richard and Patricia as well. He continued to visit the Hembroughs long after it ceased to be a financial necessity. His weekly visits are as reliable as the trains that roar past the Hembroughs' home several times each daylight hour. He described what Richard had been like before receiving GDNF.

"The biggest thing I saw was the lack of confidence to do anything. Once the confidence goes, it's a hell of a fight to get it back again. But on taking the drug, that seemed to flow back in again. It was quite incredible. I could see the progress on a weekly basis, how he was improving. Once he was on the drug and it was working, he was looking to the future in an optimistic way. It was remarkable, the change that went on."

Parkinson's had made Richard an old man before he had yet reached middle age; and, though GDNF didn't go so far as to return him to his youth, it did give back to him a few of the productive, middle-aged years Parkinson's had exacted. He had witnessed his own body's slow rebellion. His body and self had drifted apart over the years like estranged twins.

This began to change during the three years Richard spent on GDNF. The drug seemed to reconcile Richard's will with that of his body, bringing them together to make amends after the decades-old feud. It was a feeling of oneness Richard hadn't experienced since his early childhood in Warmley.

"I felt like everything was coming together," he said. "I was becoming whole as a person."

13 Word Gets Out

Richard's improvements were extraordinary. They were also common among the other Bristol patients. Their average off-medication motor score dropped from just under 35 to around 15.[20] Dr. Gill later said that he was surprised not only by the magnitude of the improvements but also by how quickly they occurred:

> By about three months we were pretty astonished at the changes that happened, not only in the motor activity, but also in the patients' motivation and drive. They looked different: their faces looked younger, more animated, and actually had a sparkle in their eyes. They were able to do things that they weren't capable of doing on their own—decorating houses, being active, taking on things they had previously been able to do. . . . There were quite dramatic changes there. And they just went on and on and on getting better.

When Dr. Gill announced the preliminary results of his trial at a meeting of the American Academy of Neurology in Denver in

April of 2002, the small clinic at Frenchay Hospital was unprepared for the deluge of media coverage that would follow. BBC Radio aired an interview with Dr. Gill and a report from Reuters appeared in major newspapers in the United States and the U.K.

"We thought that this drug would take some months or even years to be effective. We found that within a month or two patients were noticing significant changes in their ability to do things," Dr. Gill told the BBC.[21] He was careful to note that the five patients in Bristol were part of a preliminary trial, and that GDNF would need to go through additional tests before it would reach the commercial market. Nevertheless, Dr. Gill's office was flooded with requests from patients from all over the world—sufferers of Parkinson's, stroke, Alzheimer's, ALS and other disorders. GDNF was now a drug to watch in the Parkinson's pipeline.

By the time news of the Bristol trial broke, a second phase I trial was just starting at the University of Kentucky in Lexington. The Kentucky doctors finally had received approval from the FDA to move forward with the trial, and they began admitting subjects into the study in May of 2002. The principal investigator of the Kentucky trial was John Slevin, a neurology professor and the director of the university's Movement Disorder Clinic. He joined the faculty in 1981 after a fellowship at Johns Hopkins in Baltimore. Dr. Slevin is an active, wiry man of average height. He has a gray crop of hair that often goes unkempt as he darts from office to clinic to classroom.

In designing the trial, he worked closely with Don Gash, the man who had first tested GDNF in primates back in the Synergen days. Dr. Slevin also worked with another University of Kentucky neurologist named Greg Gerhardt, a longtime supporter of GDNF research, and with a seasoned neurosurgeon named Byron Young.

For the Kentucky trial, the doctors used a pump-and-catheter system that was similar to the Bristol trial but that differed in important ways. Rather than use Dr. Gill's catheter or design one of their own, the Kentucky doctors opted for one made by Medtronic, the same device company that manufactured the pumps used in Bristol. The catheter had an outer diameter of 1.65 mm compared with Dr. Gill's .6-mm invention. And while the Bristol catheter had a single hole, or port, through which the GDNF was dispensed, the catheter that the Kentucky doctors chose had 40 holes along its tip. The multi-port catheter would deliver GDNF as a soaker hose waters a garden, through dozens of perforations in its side.

The FDA required that the new pump-and-catheter system be tested in monkeys, and once it had proven safe the Kentucky doctors began to admit patients into the study. Amgen initially had declined to finance the trial, but, when the dramatic results from the Bristol trial were published, Amgen offered to take over as the Kentucky trial's sponsor. Amgen therefore would finance the trial and would submit the necessary reports to the FDA. The Kentucky doctors had begun on a shoestring: they had only enough funding for the first two patients and would have had to come up with additional funds as the trial progressed. They accepted Amgen's offer gladly, and the company assumed the role of trial sponsor in September of 2002.

Eight men and two women enrolled, and each was implanted with a single pump, tube and catheter. Parkinson's symptoms tend to be dominant on one side of the body, and, like Henry Webb in Bristol, the Kentucky patients would receive GDNF in the side of the brain opposite the most afflicted side of the body.

The FDA required that the patients be started on the low dose of 3 μg (micrograms, or millionths of a gram) a day. After eight weeks the dose would increase to 10 μg a day and then to 30 μg a day after another eight weeks. As in the Bristol trial, the chief goal of the Kentucky trial was to show that GDNF could be delivered safely. As Dr. Gill had done in Bristol, however, the Kentucky doctors assessed the patients at regular intervals to see whether the drug eased their Parkinson's symptoms. What they observed confirmed their belief in the drug's potential.

14 Case #3: Roger Thacker

Roger Thacker was seventh of the 10 patients who joined the GDNF trial in Kentucky. He claims a "normal childhood, normal life," but he was born in England and came to Kentucky by way of Africa, reminding one how relative a term is "normal." As a boy he lived in Northern England, and during World War II rode out the conflict at his uncle's farm in the Lake District of Derbyshire. He remembers a sky crammed with British and American bombers flying southeast to the Continent by the hundreds like noisy migratory birds. After the war, when Roger was eight years old, his father moved the family to Cape Town, South Africa. His father invested in hotels and farming, and Roger was exposed to both enterprises in his youth.

He grew to love animals. During a school trip, he came across an injured falcon that lay in the dust on the side of the road. He put it in a box and took it home with him. He kept the bird in a shed on his father's property and nursed it back to health. In England and in Africa, Roger had observed the sport of falconry, in which a trained bird of prey is used to hunt small game. He had seen the falconer men with birds perched on their arms, the birds' powerful feet bound with leather straps. Roger found a length of leather and imitated what he had seen. Over the course of one month, he fed the bird and taught it to fly. One day the falcon flew away and did not return. Roger remained an avid falconer throughout his life until Parkinson's made it impossible. For 12 years he would serve as president of the North American Falconry Association, and he was made an honorary member of similar associations in England and Germany.

At age 17, Roger returned to London to study agriculture and business administration at the Berkshire College of Agriculture. Upon graduation he began a career of managing animal research facilities at major universities. At the invitation of an American colleague he left London to manage the facility at Ohio State University. He later worked in similar roles at the University of Connecticut and at a private facility in Tacoma, Washington, before being recruited to the University of Kentucky in Lexington.

Roger was tall and distinguished. His mother had been a very proper, very "British" woman, he later said, and Roger's public persona projected her polished English decorum. From his father he inherited a tenacious work ethic. No sooner would he return from the university in the evenings than he was out tending sheep, mending fences and cutting or bailing hay on a 52-acre farm he had purchased just southwest of Lexington.

Roger met Linda on a blind dinner date in December of 1988. She was smart, feisty, and funny and a devout Mormon. She was more than a foot shorter than Roger, yet her energy and zeal seemed to make up all of the difference. The couple courted for three years and married in June of 1991, and Linda joined Roger on his farm.

Roger's first encounter with GDNF probably occurred without his knowledge. In the mid-1990s, Don Gash at the University of Kentucky was conducting the first primate tests of GDNF for Synergen, in the days before Amgen acquired the rights to GDNF. Roger oversaw the care of the primates used in those first tests, though Roger's was an administrative role, and he had little or no direct interaction with the GDNF-treated monkeys. At the time, he had not been diagnosed with Parkinson's and could not have imagined that the experimental drug that was being tested in his animals would eventually course through the cells of his own brain.

In the late 1990s, Roger began to walk with a slight limp and noticed a shaking in his right hand. He went to an orthopedic doctor for an examination, and after completing some tests asked the doctor, "Will I be walking normally again?"

"No," the doctor replied. "You have Parkinson's."

A neurologist's formal diagnosis confirmed that assessment in early 1998. Roger thought of his late father, who in his sixties began to suffer bodily tremor. The man never spoke of having Parkinson's, but as the disease progressed in Roger, he recognized in himself the symptoms he had observed years earlier in his father. Roger's own disease advanced briskly; the symptoms seemed to grow more severe by the day. Roger's toes began to point skyward as the muscles in his foot tightened to lift the digits unnaturally aloft. Wearing shoes became too painful, and he began to wear socks with sandals to work. The tremor in his right hand, which had begun as a gentle rolling of the thumb and forefinger, had amplified to a full-arm shake.

Within only three years of his diagnosis, Roger was in an advanced stage of the disease. In addition to the curled-up toes, the tremor, and a developing Parkinson's mask, he seemed particularly prone to painful bouts of rigidity. The muscles of his legs, arms, or trunk would seize up and remain flexed for hours. Roger in those moments was a teetering statue. To feed him, Linda literally would tie him to a chair to keep him upright. For the soreness in his muscles, Linda applied a topical pain cream continuously. She would use one $4 tube each day, and an $8 box of pain-relief patches every other day. The cost would have amounted to $243 a month.

The disease isolated Roger in myriad ways. It weakened his voice and slurred his speech. It masked his face with a permanent look of apathy. Friends and colleagues began to avoid him because he looked entirely disinterested. Parkinson's also made Roger sensitive to loud noises and general commotion, which made visits from grandchildren especially unpleasant.

It was during this advanced stage of Parkinson's that Roger first beheld the lady in gray. She was a small woman, slightly bowed, with a flowing gray cape with a hood that obscured her face. Sometimes she came alone, and sometimes she brought children, but Roger could never see her face. Roger knew the lady in gray was a hallucination—the result of one of the many pills he swallowed each day. Her visits were nonetheless comforting because Roger sensed that the lady in gray knew his pain and frustration, perhaps because she suffered from Parkinson's or some other illness.

In early 2003, Dr. Slevin told Roger and Linda about the GDNF trial. Roger said the Kentucky doctors and nurses were very straightforward about the risks. "It would be successful, we would die, or we would come out as idiots," he said of his prospects going in. Nevertheless, he later said, he felt the disease left him little choice in the matter. He would participate in the study for three reasons: "One, to improve my own situation; two, for my children's sake, hoping for some cure; and three, for the general public. Nobody ought to have to suffer and to go through this."

His surgery took place in November of 2003.

Course on GDNF

Roger had received GDNF for about two months when he noticed something different about his feet: "I looked down one morning, and I said, 'Linda, my toes have gone down!'"

It was true. Linda could see that Roger's toes were more horizontal than vertical. Roger was able to wear shoes for the first time in two years. Soon after, Roger's features began to soften as the unnatural mask gave way to a native expressiveness. Linda recalled: "We went to the hospital for one of his visits and the nurse said, 'I see we don't have a mask today.'"

Aches and pains began to subside. The freezing and the rigidity occurred less and less frequently. Roger said the improvements came gradually with noticeable milestones. "After I'd been on it six months, it was wonderful," he said. "After the full year, I was able to get on a tractor and my combines and cut hay."

Linda found that she was spending less time and money on the pain ointment and patches. "Before GDNF, he was literally being wrapped like a mummy in the patches," she said. "A year into the study, I didn't even buy them anymore."

Roger required a wheelchair for his first few visits to the hospital to have the pump refilled. "But," Linda said, "by the end of the 11 months he was on the drug, he was walking in and walking out."

Roger continued to take his other medications, including the common dopamine-replacement drug Sinemet, at the same levels he had before the study. After six months or so on GDNF, Roger began to experience the dyskinesia typical of a patient who is overmedicated. Dr. Slevin told Roger he might benefit by decreasing his dose of Sinemet. To the Thackers, this change was significant because it suggested to them that Roger's natural dopamine levels were increasing, which meant GDNF might very well be reviving Roger's withered brain cells.

Every two months during the trial, a nurse would give Roger a UPDRS assessment, as had been done in Bristol. His off-medication motor score was 34 when he started the trial. After six months, the score had dropped to just above 20. His on-medication score dropped from near 20 to below 5. In essence, the numbers show that Roger's best of days before the GDNF trial were about the same as his worst of days after it. And after six months on GDNF, Roger was very close to normal during his "on" times.[22]

"It wasn't like he didn't have Parkinson's anymore," Linda said. "He still had his 'off' times. But it was just becoming more doable. I could leave for four hours at a time, and I knew he would be fine. And there were *some* big changes. Just a month or two before the drug was taken away, Roger got down on the floor and played with the grandchildren. That was just the most exciting thing. We just stood and watched him."

15 Amgen's Phase II Trial

After the success of the Bristol trial and as the Kentucky trial was getting underway, Amgen sent one if its neurologists, a British-born scientist named Michael Traub, to Bristol to interview the doctors and patients there. When he returned, he too was convinced of GDNF's potential, and Dr. Traub remained a staunch advocate within Amgen for the development of GDNF.

Dan Lee, an Amgen employee who worked closely with GDNF from the time Amgen acquired rights to it in 1994, said Dr. Traub was a thin man of average height and in his early 60s who was usually disheveled and always brilliant:

> He wasn't a typical corporate. He was very anti-corporate, and he wouldn't tolerate any stupidity. He was demanding and he was sarcastic if you weren't on the right track. You had to be on your toes. He was a good guy and he was honest. He was very smart and usually ahead of most people. His hair was always messed up, and if he shaved, he would miss patches. He would dress casually. He would drink

> really strong coffee all morning—he drank a lot of coffee and he fidgeted a lot. But when he set his mind to writing and saying something that was difficult and required thought, he was brilliant.

On Dr. Traub's recommendation and on the strength of the Bristol study, Amgen, in early 2003, launched a third clinical trial, its largest and most scientifically rigorous to date. Dr. Traub called on a half-dozen distinguished clinicians in the Parkinson's research field to design the protocol for the trial. Unlike the Bristol and Kentucky trials, which had been phase I trials and primarily designed to test for safety, this trial would be a phase II trial and would be designed to test whether GDNF was effective.

Amgen patterned the phase II trial after the trial in Bristol. Each patient would have pumps and catheters implanted on both sides of the body. There was some discussion about what would be an appropriate dose. The Bristol patients' dose had not been constant: Dr. Gill had gradually increased it from 14 μg a day (per pump) to 45 μg a day and back down again, amounting to an overall per-patient average of about 25 μg a day. Because the Bristol patients had improved significantly even on the lower dose, Amgen decided on a dose of 15 μg a day per pump for the phase II study. The trial would involve 34 patients at seven sites around the world—five sites in the United States, one in Canada, and one in England.[23]

The clinicians that Amgen consulted disagreed over what type of catheter should be used for the phase II trial. Dr. Gill had taken great pains in designing a slim catheter that would fit snugly in the brain, allowing him to deliver the drug under pressure through convection-enhanced delivery. However, some of the clinicians doubted it was necessary to force the drug into the tissue. In any case, Dr. Gill's catheter hadn't been approved for clinical use by the FDA, and getting the approval would delay the start of the trial.

Amgen opted for a Medtronic catheter that was 1 mm thick. The stainless steel guide tube used to insert it was 1.7 mm thick, which meant that a channel of .7 mm would be left around the catheter after the guide tube was removed. The company also elected not to use convection enhanced delivery, according to Dr. Gill's model. The GDNF would be dripped, rather than pushed, into the *putamen*.

Dr. Gill protested, as did Clive Svendsen, a neurologist from the University of Wisconsin-Madison who had worked with Dr. Gill on the Bristol trial. But Dr. Gill said he worried about advocating for his catheter too forcefully, since taking such a stance likely would be viewed as self-interested.

"Obviously I wanted my catheter used," he later said. "I had at that point patented the catheter, but I couldn't stand and shout because people would think, 'Well, he only wants it because it's his catheter.' I did make noise, though. And Clive Svendsen made noise."

A profile of Dr. Svendsen in the July 2004 issue of the journal *Nature Medicine*, reports that he "fell out" with Amgen during these negotiations: "The problem was Amgen's proposed methodology, says Svendsen. The company wanted to use thicker—and potentially more damaging—catheters. It also wanted to enroll 34 mid- to late-stage study subjects, but Svendsen argued that such patients probably have very few dopamine neurons left to save, reducing GDNF's chances of success."

Svendsen refused to take part in the trial under conditions that, in his mind, were setting the trial up for failure. Dr. Gill stayed on and became one of seven lead investigators for the multi-center phase II trial. In addition to his first five patients, who continued to receive GDNF, he would enlist 10 new subjects for the phase II trial. Neurologists at the various sites recruited patients to the trial throughout 2003. The volunteers had to be between 35 and 70 years old and had to have been diagnosed at least five years prior. The primary goal or "endpoint" in this trial was a 25 percent improvement in the patients' motor scores.[24]

All 34 of the patients in Amgen's phase II trial underwent surgery and were implanted with two pumps—one for each side of the brain, as in the Bristol trial. But only 17 of the patients were given GDNF during the six-month study. The other 17 received a saline placebo. The trial was double-blinded, so neither the patients nor the doctors knew who got GDNF and who the saline placebo.

The trial was carried out at Frenchay Hospital in Bristol and at medical centers at the University of Kentucky, the University of Virginia, the University of Toronto, the University of Chicago, New York University, Duke University in Durham, N.C., and Oregon Health and Science University in Portland. The number of patients at each of the sites varied—from as many as 10 in Bristol to as few as three at Chicago, Duke, and NYU.

At each site, a lead investigator oversaw the trial and made sure it followed a detailed protocol that Amgen had drafted. The lead investigators at the sites were not Amgen employees. Most of them were faculty members of the universities and had distinguished careers as neurologists and neurosurgeons.

By the time the phase II trial got underway, the Parkinson's patient community was looking to GDNF as the most promising treatment to surface since the advent of L-dopa. Not uncommonly, a Parkinson's patient will read about some so-called miracle drug in the pipeline, but, because no breakthrough treatment has come to market in the past 40 years, patients tend to grow skeptical of the claims. By the time GDNF entered the phase II trial, though, it had enough momentum and credibility to get the patient community's attention. Dave Heydrick, a Maryland neurologist and a Parkinson's patient himself, was following GDNF's development closely and saw the stir it caused in the Parkinson's community. "GDNF came to be seen as the last great hope," he said. "People expected it to be the silver bullet."

16 Case #4: Bob Suthers

Bob Suthers was one of three GDNF patients at the trial site at New York University. Perhaps no one gave more to the GDNF trials than Bob. He may not ever realize just how much.

In September of 2003, Bob spent six hours in a surgical suite at the New York University Medical Center as a neurosurgeon sliced open his stomach, drilled holes in his skull and installed the hardware he would carry for the next three years. Bob was recovering at the hospital the following day when his eyes rolled back and his body was overcome by the rhythmic convulsions of a grand mal seizure. Bob had suffered a stroke.

He spent the following three weeks in the hospital's intensive care unit. When he regained consciousness after the seizure, he couldn't speak, couldn't recognize family, didn't respond to his own name. His speech returned gradually; he would recover most of his mental capacity.

A skull X-ray revealed that during his seizure Bob had jarred loose the catheter on the left side of his brain. His neurologist, Michael Hutchinson, said he could either have the pumps, tubes, and catheters removed and withdraw from the trial or undergo a second surgery to have the catheter repositioned. He opted to stay in the trial and had a second surgery in mid-October of 2003. Within a few days of returning home after the second surgery, he began to feel better than he had in years.

"He was sure he had GDNF. He felt really good, like he was getting better. He got very excited," Elaine said. "But that was not long-lasting. It lasted about a week or so."

Bob didn't know it at the time, but he had been randomly assigned to the placebo arm of the trial, which meant he got an ineffective saline solution for the first six months of the study. Elaine, who had worked as a nurse in New York City for more than 35 years, said the sensation of improvement that Bob had felt was a classic placebo effect. She had seen it many times in the patients she cared for. It wasn't until the six-month study had ended and Amgen gave GDNF to all of the phase II patients that she saw Bob begin to make real improvements.

Bob's early life is better documented than that of any other GDNF patient I interviewed. After retirement, he wrote his personal history and eventually had it published and bound in a volume he titled *Journey: The quest to finding myself.*

In the introduction, Bob writes: "The major part of this book is about my first 33 years . . . the epilogue is the next 33 years of my life in summation. I did this [because] my first 33 years were unique and interesting. The second 33 years were interesting but not unique." Bob wrote the autobiography in 2002, a year before beginning the GDNF trials. Had he known where the GDNF trials would take him, he might have phrased the introduction a bit differently. His time on GDNF and the years that followed were nothing if not unique.

He was born in 1934 in upstate New York in his grandfather's farmhouse, a worn building with no electricity or running water.

Bob's mother, Claire Suthers, had traveled from Long Island to deliver the baby. She was 19 when Bob, her second child, was born. Bob's father abandoned Claire immediately after Bob's birth. She returned to Long Island with two children and few prospects. Claire's second husband provided a home for the family but not much else, and when Bob was 12 his step-father told him to start looking for a job. From that point on Bob bought his own clothes and paid his parents for room and board. He got a summer job at a nearby potato farm on what was then a rural Long Island. He labored beside migrant workers who colored his vocabulary and accelerated his already speedy transition to adulthood. He grew tall and athletic and played sports in school. He was interested in girls but was shy, brooding, and withdrawn. In his book, he refers often to an "inner rage" that went on mounting from childhood—a resentment toward the men in his life who had let him down. As a boy he fought regularly at recess. As a young man, he found it hard to grow close to people.

Bob joined the Army at 18 and spent almost two years in Okinawa, Japan in the mid-1950s. He had long been a devout Catholic, and when he returned from Japan, Bob began to seriously consider entering a monastery. In the fall of 1957, he began as six-month postulancy at a monastery in Pittsburg—a sort of apprenticeship to determine whether monastic life suited him. For 12 years it did, and Bob spent most of that time at the Holy Family Monastery in West Hartford, Connecticut. While at Holy Family he attended a class on nursing taught by a pretty young nun at a convent for the Sisters of Mercy. She was introduced as Sister Mary-Hope. Her birth name was Elaine Rasoft.

Four years later, when Bob told Sister Mary-Hope that he planned to leave the monastery and return to secular life, she replied that she, too, had considered leaving the convent. The two married in 1968 and made their home in Greenlawn, the town where Bob had grown up. They had three daughters: Mary, Hope and Kristen.

Bob's "interesting but not unique" period was spent working for a New York-based textile company called J.P. Stevens during the following 29 years. Elaine got a job at NYU's Medical Center. Bob remained active and athletic and in 1990 ran the New York Marathon. He retired from J.P. Stevens in 1997.

Elaine first noticed the tremor in Bob's hand as they sat at lunch one day in Huntington Village Diner about four miles from their home in Greenlawn: "He was talking away and he didn't seem to be aware of it. I saw the tremor then and a few times after that, but I kept denying it. Several months later, I was talking to my gynecologist, and she asked how Bob was doing. I told her about Bob's tremors, and she said, "Elaine, he has Parkinson's.' And I said, 'I know,' and I burst into tears. I was a nurse. I knew Parkinson's. But I was in denial."

Bob was diagnosed with Parkinson's in 1998 by Dr. Gobindan Gopinathan at the NYU Medical Center and soon after became the patient of Michael Hutchinson. Bob took the news hard. "I felt devastated. I had known a priest in the monastery who had Parkinson's disease. That was before the days of L-dopa, and I saw how he was and thought that's how I was going to become. I was depressed for a while, but I managed to get over it. I went on with regular life."

Bob's symptoms progressed quickly. He said Dr. Hutchinson "tried almost every combination" of available medication, but by 2002, Bob was quickly becoming immobile. He and Elaine could no longer walk the few blocks into the town center for lunch or to shop. He sat at home most of every day. His "on" times diminished to less than two hours, with "off" times at least that long in between.

A Parkinson's-induced mask began to deaden Bob's ordinarily expressive, easy smile. It made him appear bored and uninterested; and he found that the mask, combined with his other symptoms, scared off neighbors, friends, and relatives from visiting him at home. A profound loneliness set in, and Bob became frustrated and despondent. His outlet was writing, but after some months, Parkinson's robbed him of that, too. His handwritten script degenerated into a tiny, cramped, indecipherable scrawl.

Bob wasn't interested when Dr. Hutchinson first mentioned the GDNF trials. "Bob's words were, 'Nobody's ever going to drill a hole in my head,'" Elaine recalled. She had her own reservations about the invasive surgery. "I really didn't want him to have it done —but I didn't tell him that. Then one day we went out to lunch with Hope and Kristen, and Bob announced he was going to have the surgery. I was surprised, and I was worried, but I knew it was his last chance at normalcy."

Elaine said she remembers asking Dr. Hutchinson what would happen if Amgen decided to stop developing GDNF. "When I worried about them taking it away, Dr. Hutchinson said, 'Why would they take it away from you if it works?'"

Though he once scoffed at the idea of having holes drilled into his skull, Bob gradually became realistic about the futility of not doing so. "I knew there was no cure. I knew my symptoms were getting worse," he said. "And it seemed like it [the GDNF trial] was coming from a responsible company."

Bob underwent several hours of testing—first to determine whether he qualified for the study and later to gauge his mobility for a before-and-after comparison. The first surgery took place on September 9, 2003. After the stroke, Bob underwent the second surgery on October 16. For six months, his brain was doused with a steady trickle of a saline placebo. On March 30, 2004, Bob had GDNF pumped into his brain for the first time.

Course on GDNF

Because of Bob's previous experience with the placebo effect, Bob and Elaine were more cautious when Bob started on GDNF. It wasn't as if Bob had imagined those improvements—he really had felt better during the first two weeks on placebo. The false alarm made them wary about attributing too much to GDNF, but they remained hopeful.

The improvements Bob felt on GDNF were neither immediate nor particularly pronounced. "The improvement couldn't be seen during the first month or so," Bob said. "It was very gradual."

Each month Bob and Elaine would make their way to the NYU Medical Center for a refilling of the pump. Bob was too weak and unsteady to make the trip by train; his legs would give out on the walk across Penn Station to the subway. So each month the couple would pay $375 for a car service to pick them up from home, deposit them at the entrance of the NYU Medical Center, and then wait for the return trip home. During the first six months of the trial, while Bob was on the placebo but didn't know it, they used the car service.

In May of 2004, after he had been on GDNF for two months, Bob told Elaine that he felt strong and steady enough to take the train. Elaine protested, but Bob insisted. He remembers the trip this way: "I walked from the parking lot to the station and I was feeling fine. We took the train to Penn Station, and when we got there, we walked across Penn Station to the subway line that runs over to NYU. We took the bus along 34th Street, and then we walked from there to the medical center. When I walked through those doors, the nurses must have had no idea why I was smiling so big. I don't think I could have explained it to them, either."

The victory was small but intensely meaningful for Bob. All he had known of Parkinson's was weakening, regression, backsliding, and loss. The successful trip to the city (and back!) was evidence that the disease was not unassailable. It was like turning back the tide—miraculous, even if only turned back an inch.

The improvements continued during the summer of 2004. Bob's legs felt increasingly steady beneath him, and he resumed his walks into Greenlawn for lunch with Elaine. He could concentrate better, and he could sit and read the morning paper, as before. Bob said his confidence and his energy seemed to increase by the day. After several months on GDNF, he began to cut back on his other medication—sometimes he would skip doses even though he wasn't supposed to. He regained his ability to write.

By sheer coincidence, all three of Dr. Hutchinson's patients had been randomized into the placebo group during the original six-month trial. Dr. Hutchinson later said he observed no lasting improvements until the study had ended and each of the patients was given GDNF. At that point, he said, Bob, a woman named Niwana Martin, and a third patient each showed clear improvements.

"Bob stopped tremoring and was walking briskly and gracefully, Niwana Martin went back to horseback riding and kayaking, and there was a third patient who also improved," Dr. Hutchinson said. "You could literally see the difference in these patients from one visit to the next."

For Bob and Elaine, who remained religious throughout their lives, Bob's recovery was a miracle—perhaps a recompense for the dozen years both had spent in the Lord's service.

17 Case #5: Steve Kaufman

Steve Kaufman was the first GDNF patient I ever met. We were introduced at the World Parkinson's Congress in Washington D.C., and my interview with him was influential in my decision to take on the book project. He joined Amgen's phase II trial at the site in Chicago.

He was born in September of 1954 to Wayne and Rosie Kaufman in Evanston, Illinois. Steve spent each summer of his childhood at his grandfather's cabin in northern Wisconsin. It was a sturdy, Finnish-style structure at the end of a winding, seven-mile dirt road. Steve grew up in Chicago's suburbs, and the 18-acre plot of forest was his connection to a world that had long been paved over back home.

Steve's mother died when he was 6 years old, and family members and neighbors encouraged Wayne to put Steve and his younger sister up for adoption. Steve later said that "back then, that was the way people thought—men didn't raise kids. He said, 'I'm not having any part of that. These are my kids and I'm going to raise them. And if you guys don't like that, you can go to Hell!'"

Wayne was a hefty, gruff man whom the neighborhood children would call "Fred Flintstone." It was an apt comparison, Steve admits, because though he was stern and prone to raise his voice, he was also a dedicated family man who loved his children and raised them well. Wayne worked as a deliveryman for a lumber yard, and the company allowed him to sit the children in the cab of the truck during the summer months when they weren't in school. Eventually he remarried, and Steve said his stepmother, Joyce, raised him and his sister as if they were her own.

Steve says his mother's death left a void and a nagging need for attachment. He spent the summer of his tenth year, as usual, at the cabin. His grandfather had built the cabin in the 1940s, and the family had made friends with the residents of nearby Mercer, a small town 40 miles or so south of Lake Superior. One of his grandfather's friends was a man named Vernon Blank who would have been in his late forties when Steve was a boy. He was of average height and build, and he was the man Steve's family would call when something broke. He didn't seem to mind Steve hanging by his side and watching him work.

The cabin's water came from a shallow well, and one day the electric pump broke, so the family called Vernon. The pump was underground in a cramped, cinderblock-lined pit about seven feet deep. Vernon surmised that the hole was too narrow for a man and that Steve would have to be lowered in to replace a faulty valve. Steve recalls being terrified: "He said, 'Okay, you're going down and you're going to replace this valve.' I really didn't want to go down there and he said, 'There's nothing to be afraid of. There's nothing down there. It's just a dark damp hole.' I went down there; he lowered me down into it. There were spider webs, and I was imagining these spiders with monster fangs. I was scared, but when I got done, and he pulled me out, I had replaced the valve and the pump worked! It changed my whole attitude from that point on. I knew I could do certain things . . . I kind of clung to him, and he started showing me how to fix things, even at a young age. He kind of planted the seed in me, saying, 'Just about everything is fixable, but you gotta look at it in a reasonable manner.'"

Steve continued to fix and build things throughout his youth and adulthood. With some neighborhood friends he built a go-kart, and Steve discovered that another of his passions was speed. Steve came to love speedboats, downhill skiing and any other activity that would send the wind whistling through his hair. When he was 16, his father cosigned on a loan for a car—a 1970 Oldsmobile 442 W30. It was red, it was fast, and it made his stepmother furious when the boys brought it home. "It said 'race' all over it," Steve remembered. "She didn't talk to Dad for two weeks."

Steve met Maggie at a party when he was 18. She had sneaked out from a friend's house to be there and looked apprehensive where she sat alone on a couch. Steve walked over and introduced himself. Maggie was pretty, intelligent, and shy. The conversation was pleasant but short—Maggie was getting nervous about her parents and had to go. Steve wouldn't see her again for another 10 years.

After college, Steve took a new job at a distribution center, and Maggie hired on with the same company a short time later. It wasn't until they had dated several times that the couple realized they had met at a party back in high school. Now, both had been married and divorced. Neither was anxious to make another mistake, so they courted each other with caution. Maggie had shed her youthful shyness and was talkative, spontaneous, and a fine match for Steve. They dated seriously for 18 months and were married in June of 1984.

The Kaufmans moved several times but stayed in the Chicago area. Steve eventually took a job at a distribution center for Canon Inc., and Maggie began working for a metal products manufacturing company. The couple continued to make trips to the cabin up north and kept in touch with Vernon and his wife Lillian. Eventually, Maggie and Steve bought a Northern Wisconsin property of their own.

In 1991, Steve's father was diagnosed with Parkinson's, at age 64. Wayne had never been one to give up easily, but in Parkinson's he saw something insurmountable, Steve said. "He was always a fighter, but for some reason, he just gave up on this. He was a big guy, a strong guy, but when he started noticing the tremors and he started losing weight . . . he started realizing he couldn't do certain things, and it just demoralized him. . . . I told him, 'Dad, you can fight this.'

"But he said, 'No, there's no cure.'

"I said, 'There's always faith and hope, you've just got to say your prayers, and just fight it.'

"But he said, 'No, I'm a dead man.'

"It just took hold of him right away. He just gave up."

Within a few years of his father's diagnosis, Steve learned that Vernon, his childhood mentor and longtime friend, also had been diagnosed with the disease. The two most significant male figures in his life had been afflicted with the same disease. Steve's own diagnosis followed by only a few years.

Steve believes that exposure to pesticides in his youth brought on his Parkinson's. Until the early 1970s, when it was banned, the pesticide DDT was a staple for repelling mosquitoes. At the cabin, Steve's grandfather had rigged a lawnmower so that it functioned as a mosquito fogger. The machine's blade had been removed and an extra gas tank had been bolted onto the engine. Steve's grandfather showed him how to fill that tank, half with water, half with a clear liquid from a red and yellow bottle. A copper tube connected the extra tank to the motor's exhaust port, and once started, the contraption puffed a steady plume of white smoke that hung in the air as Steve maneuvered around the perimeter of the cabin's backyard.

When the tank would run dry, Steve would fetch the red and yellow bottle, whose label warned to "Wash hands after handling!" He would sometimes spill the liquid on his fingers. So, heeding the bottle's warning, he would quickly wash his hands the way most boys would: by wiping them vigorously on his blue jeans. Both Steve and his father had fairly regular exposure to DDT, which studies have since linked to the disease.[25] He was 40 when he learned he had Parkinson's.

Steve was diagnosed in January of 1995, and the disease progressed quickly. It weakened his ankles, buckled his legs, slurred his speech, and slowed his life to a pace excruciating for a man with a passion for speed. His father's progression advanced a few years ahead of his own. Eventually, Wayne could no longer be cared for at home and moved into an assisted living center.

"We would go and see him as much as we could," Steve said. "I didn't go as much as I should have, and the reason why was [that] I was seeing how he was spiraling downward, and it was like looking at a mirror. I was thinking, 'Oh boy, is this what I'm going to be looking at in a couple of years?' He understood why I didn't come there all the time."

Eight years after his diagnosis, Steve was, according to his neurologist, "maxed out" on his current medications. He had given up his favorite pastimes of fishing, downhill skiing, and boating. He slept a fitful hour or two each night, which left him exhausted and dozing at work during the day. Steve had a reputation among his neighbors as an able mechanic, and when they would come to him with car trouble, he was increasingly unable to help. "I would tell them, 'Well, I can look at it, and I can guide you, but I can't do any of the work myself.' My hands just weren't steady enough."

He made an appointment to see Dr. Arif Dalvi at the University of Chicago Medical Center. Dr. Dalvi administered several tests to determine whether Deep Brain Stimulation was a good choice for Steve. He spoke with Steve during the examination, and Steve remembered the conversation this way:

"At that halfway point, he said to me, 'You know, DBS is basically like a Band-Aid. In some cases it will stop the tremors, but it's not going to stop dyskinesia. It's not going to stop you from falling—you're going to fall. It's going to stop the tremors—that's all it really does. It's not going to lessen the rigidity. But on the other hand, we've got this new trial that's about to [begin] called GDNF, have you heard of it?'"

Steve was surprised by the coincidence. He had read about GDNF on the Internet the night before. He told Dr. Dalvi that he didn't know much about it, but that it sounded promising. Steve recalls that Dr. Dalvi said, "Well, we are a center for this study, and I think you would be a good candidate for it. Are you interested?"

Maggie was in the room, and Steve could see right away that she was not interested. She hadn't been fond of DBS, a proven treatment that had been given successfully to thousands of patients worldwide. GDNF was a shot in the dark by comparison, tested successfully in only 15 humans. She seemed to bristle when Steve expressed interest in the trial. Dr. Dalvi asked Steve to think about the trial during the next two weeks. Steve said he would consider it, and the couple made their way to the car.

"It was the quietest ride home," Steve later said. "Not a word was said between the two of us. We were about ten miles from the house when I finally said, 'Well, what do you think?' She just broke into tears.

"I'm scared," Steve recalled Maggie saying. "I'm not happy with either way you're going to choose. But on the flip side, knowing you, you already made up your mind."

"Yeah, I did," Steve answered.

"What are you thinking?" she asked him.

"I'm thinking about going with the GDNF."

"Why?"

"Well, I think I could benefit mankind. I think I could definitely be a help to mankind."

"Why would you think that?"

"I don't know," Steve said. "I feel very strongly about it. I read about it on the Internet and it showed very promising results. I think that I might get on this bandwagon, and if it works for me like I'm reading, we could cure this thing.'"

Vernon Blank had taught Steve that any problem could be solved if it was approached in the right way. Maybe GDNF was the way to solve Parkinson's. Steve underwent the surgery on November 13, 2003. He was randomly assigned to receive GDNF, and he got the drug continuously for the following nine months.

Course on GDNF

The Kaufmans live in the verdant Chicago suburb of Algonquin. Behind the house is a wooden deck that, truth be told, looks like it was built by a man who felt he had something to prove.

It is a sprawling, elegant, three-tiered thing with wide platforms and a pair of staircases descending to opposite corners of the back yard. Along the deck's perimeter is a waist-high railing, with white rails capped with carved, natural wood planks. Steve Kaufman began building the deck in the summer of 2004 and finished it in November of that year. It was his second major remodeling project since starting GDNF. For the Kaufmans, the deck symbolizes what Steve had lost and what GDNF had returned to him.

After the surgery, weeks passed and Steve did not notice any changes. He continued to sleep fitfully and arrive from work exhausted.

"I noticed the first change six weeks after I got the first injection. I used to have a frown or a scowl. People used to think I was always mad. I wasn't. The Parkinson's was causing my muscles to tighten. But I was noticing that my muscles were relaxing.

"I was shaving in the morning and I realized, 'Wait a minute, I don't have this funny look any more.' I asked Maggie, 'Do you notice a change? Do you notice anything different about me?' She said, 'Yes! Your frown is disappearing!'"

At his second trip to the hospital for refilling of the pumps, Dr. Dalvi asked Steve if he had noticed any changes.

"I told him about my face muscles relaxing. And I was starting to get flexibility back in my fingers. I said, 'Look what I can do with my fingers now.'

"He said, 'That's interesting.'

"He [Dr. Dalvi] really didn't become a believer until probably the fourth month. He said to Maggie, 'I think we hit on something here. I'm looking at a totally different person than I saw a year ago.'"

By that time, Steve—the new Steve—was well into a kitchen remodeling project. He knew Maggie didn't care for the outdated cupboards that came with the house. He would have replaced them when the couple moved in, had he been able. But Parkinson's had left him without the strength or the motor control to undertake such a project. After three months on GDNF, Steve didn't feel nearly as tired after the workday. His hands and legs were steadier, too, and one day he decided he was equal to the task. Over the next two months, Steve replaced the cupboards and countertops and the kitchen sink.

Even before he finished the kitchen, Steve was imagining plans for a deck in the backyard. Prior to the GDNF trials, he couldn't even hold a nail steady, and this deck would have been a challenge even for one unencumbered by Parkinson's. Steve spent six months building the structure. He would work on it in the evenings during the week and all day on the weekends. A friend helped him place the main support beams in the ground and secure them with concrete. Then he was on his own to do the rest.

No one ever told Steve how he fared on the motor score assessments that he underwent periodically. But Steve didn't really care. It was just a number, after all, and meant little to him compared with the obvious changes he was observing in almost every aspect of his life.

"It was a great feeling," he later said. "I was improving day by day, and that was good for me. But the way I looked at it, it was also a good thing for my dad and for mankind in general. I felt like I was part of something that was going to help millions of people who have Parkinson's. It was like I was part of finding the cure."

17 Sudden Death

Dr. Mickey Traub, the Amgen scientist who had visited Bristol and had become a champion for GDNF within the company, died abruptly of a heart attack in February of 2004. He died at work at Amgen's headquarters in Thousand Oaks, midway through the phase II trial. Dr. Traub had hired a neurologist named Donna Masterman in 2003 to work on the GDNF team. Prior to that, Dr. Masterman was an assistant clinical professor of neurology at the University of California, Los Angeles, and while at UCLA she had been an investigator for the original GDNF trials, in which GDNF was injected into the ventricles of the brain. (These were the trials that were halted early because of a host of negative side effects and no significant improvements in the patients.) Dr. Masterman was Dr. Traub's presumptive replacement, and after his death, she took over lead of the phase II trial that was still in progress.

By this time, the studies in Bristol and Kentucky had ended, but the 15 patients had been given the option to continue receiving GDNF in an open-label extension of the trial. All 15 elected to do so. The five men in Bristol and the two women and eight men in

Kentucky expected to receive GDNF in this way indefinitely, they would later say, or at least until it became available commercially. One of the women in Kentucky was forced to withdraw when the skin around the catheter in her skull began to erode. The doctors worried the wound would become infected and that the infection might travel down the catheter and into her brain. The remaining 14 patients from the two phase I studies continued to receive GDNF, and they continued to improve or at least to maintain the substantial improvements they had already experienced.

Within weeks of Dr. Traub's death, on March, 6, 2004, Amgen's Vice President of Research and Development Roger Perlmutter took the podium as the keynote speaker at the "Defining the Horizons" conference at the University of California, Santa Barbara. The event was hosted by the school's Center for Engineering Entrepreneurship and Engineering Management, and Perlmutter was to speak about innovation from the perspective of the biotechnology industry. His speech was titled, "Innovation at the Interface Between Basic Research and Clinical Medicine," and it dealt almost exclusively with the development of GDNF.

Dr. Perlmutter began the speech with a summary of the physical breakdowns that occur in the brain of a Parkinson's patient, and he described how traditional treatments did nothing to stop the progression of the disease, only to mask it.

"The approach that we have taken at Amgen, and have been taking for some time is quite different," he told the crowd. "Rather than trying to treat the signs and symptoms of Parkinson's disease by increasing how much dopamine there is, we're trying to treat the disease by giving people back the dopamine-containing neurons."[26]

Developing such a treatment had not been easy. Dr. Perlmutter spoke of the early days at Synergen and the decade of animal tests that led up to the clinical trials of GDNF in the late 1990s. When those trials failed, another company might have abandoned GDNF altogether.

"But there was something tantalizing about this, and it just seemed like it was worth going the distance and administering the material where it could do the most good, which is actually within the brain substance right down where all those nerve cells were dying. I mean, if you want to protect the nerve cells you want to make sure that the substance gets to them.

"That's the subsequent experiment—and it is an experiment—that we have pursued. I began that study shortly after I arrived at Amgen. The catheter is actually drilled down into the brain—you know you dodge the piano lessons, dodge the French and try to get it down to the right place."

There is laughter from the audience.

"It's only because this is such a horrible, grievous illness that you would even consider doing this. What I would like to do is show you some of the early clinical results."

Dr. Perlmutter was referring to the results of the phase I trials in Bristol and Kentucky. On a large white screen to his right appeared a video clip of a patient undergoing a motor score assessment. At first, the movements are laborious and strained. The next clip shows a similar assessment of the same man, taken six months after he began receiving GDNF. Now his movements are easy and brisk. His once strained features are now relaxed. The difference is stark.

"It's the same guy, except that he looks like he's ready to join the Marine Corps," Dr. Perlmutter observed. "As you can see, he still has a tremor, but he's really substantially improved here." Dr. Perlmutter then spoke of biological changes that had been observed in the brains of the Bristol patients. PET scans of the brain showed an increase of activity where the GDNF was administered. The drug appeared to be restoring the body's natural processes for the production and uptake of dopamine. It suggested that what had occurred in the Bristol patients was more than mere placebo effect.

"That persuades me that—although it's very difficult to be sure—that patients are not responding to our encouragement and saying, 'Hey, we've got a therapy that might work.' They can't change the pattern of dopamine uptake in their brains."

In conclusion, Dr. Perlmutter gave what was likely a tribute to the late Dr. Traub, who at the time had been dead only weeks. Dr. Perlmutter didn't mention his former colleague by name, but his closing remarks suggest that the man was in his thoughts.

> Innovation in biotechnology begins with exploratory research. It inevitably depends upon individual product champions. Somebody out there really believes in this thing, and they're willing to go to the mat for it time and time again. They have to because all great products die a thousand deaths en route to commercialization. They all do. I've never been associated with one . . . that didn't die and die and die and have to be resurrected constantly. So many times during the GDNF story it seemed like this would never make it—it may not make it still—but somebody had to be behind it, championing it.[27]

Dr. Traub had been such a champion for GDNF. From the time he visited Dr. Gill and the five original patients in Bristol, he remained and ardent supporter of GDNF development within Amgen. He had encouraged Amgen to assume sponsorship of the phase I trial in Kentucky and then prodded the company to embark on an ambitious phase II trial of its own. With Dr. Traub now gone, would someone else within Amgen's ranks step up and assume the role of champion?

Dr. Perlmutter ended his address and invited questions. A young man near the back of the room stood and asked how long it would take before a drug like GDNF would come to market and how much money it would make once it became marketable.

In answer to the first question, Dr. Perlmutter said, "We expect to be able to look at the initial data from the phase II studies in the middle of the summer. Let's say those data were positive. At that point, we would have to embark upon large studies. They don't have to be that large because of the nature of the illness. My guess is that we could probably complete a large study in a couple of years and registration would be pretty rapid, so we could probably be in the market from that period in, let's say, three years."

Three years. Given the date of Perlmutter's speech, in the winter of 2004, that would put the commercial launch of GDNF in early 2007. He next addressed the young man's second question. Dr. Perlmutter's response to the question of how much money a drug like GDNF would make gives some insight into how the company expected GDNF to perform financially.

> The cost of such studies is huge because you have to underwrite the cost for each patient for the neurosurgical procedure and everything else. So the cost is very, very large. At the end of the day what matters is, it comes down to perverse incentives that exist in the marketplace, so let me tell you about some of those. If we were able to succeed with this therapy and it's terrific and [there is] no long term toxicity, and it's better than anything, nerves are growing—all that kind of stuff—there aren't enough neurosurgeons in the country to do that procedure, and there aren't enough neurosurgical suites in which to do it, so that will limit you pretty dramatically. But that part, eventually you could

ramp up to that. Hospitals would much prefer to have their neurosurgeons doing surgery for lower back pain. They want quick turnover in that operating room. They prefer not to have their operating room involved in a procedure that takes many, many hours to perform and involves a huge team of trained neurosurgeons. They'd like to have a lower cost. So, hospitals will very much resist this, and they'll want their neurosurgeons to continue to do spinal surgery.

So, there's a lot of education that has to be done at the level of payers, of hospitals and et cetera. And whenever you introduce a new medicine, you actually change the practice of medicine. It's actually a decade to get much traction with that. So, that's an introduction to the response of how much money would you make on such a thing. It all depends on to what extent you can penetrate the market.

It's not clear how much you would charge for such material [as GDNF] because you want to balance this and make it accessible to the largest percentage of people who actually need it. But not so under-priced that you could never recoup your investment even in a dozen years."

This is not a therapy that from our perspective is going to be a huge money maker for Amgen. It's just—you're never going to get there. It just doesn't make sense. On the other hand, we take the view that in terms of the vision of the company, we often come to the situation where we have to decide among competing projects. Our response is that we always try to put patients and patients' needs first. And to the extent that we do that it's enormously clarifying. In this case, if we have a therapy that makes this kind of difference, we'll put that first, and ultimately depend upon our ability to demonstrate that to permit the company to go

> forward. It's nice to be in a situation where we can do that, and, because of our very strong financial base, we can; but it will be challenging from a financial perspective.

According to Dr. Perlmutter, Amgen wasn't counting on GDNF to be highly profitable for the company. According to him, the company was pressing forward with the development of the drug not because of an anticipated payoff but simply because it was the right thing to do—and Amgen was in a financial position to do it. Amgen's patent on the synthetic version of GDNF was set to expire in 2017—ten years after the anticipated commercial launch of the drug in 2007. Dr. Perlmutter said it can take at least that long for a radically different treatment to gain "much traction" in the medical community. The lengthy, complex surgery would be a hard sell to hospitals and buyers, and by the time the pump-and-catheter treatment of GDNF became mainstream (if it ever did) the company's patent would have expired. Perhaps this is what Dr. Perlmutter had in mind when he said, "You're never going to get there."

18 Perfect Storm

In the early spring of 2004, the multi-center, phase II trial was just finishing up and there were promising reports coming from the various trial sites. If the results were similar to those from Bristol and Kentucky, Amgen would want to move quickly and do the additional trials that the FDA would require. The company began to draw up a protocol for a new and larger trial. It would be a phase III trial—the next step toward getting GDNF on the market and the highest hurdle a drug company must clear when developing a drug. It would probably include a hundred patients or more instead of a few dozen.

Amgen also began working out the logistics of selling GDNF commercially. The company organized a meeting it called the "GDNF Global Commercial Team Summit" that took place in mid-June—just a week or so before the results of the phase II trial were due out. Amgen flew Stephen Waite to Rome to give a first-hand account of how GDNF had transformed his life. Amgen anticipated a worldwide launch of GDNF by 2007 at the latest, assuming the results from the phase II trial didn't disappoint. Michael Reilly, who was a co-leader of Amgen's GDNF team during the summer of 2004, said the company wanted its contacts around the world to be ready:

> That meeting is an indicator of Amgen's preparations and seriousness in launching. . . . We had moved from decisions being made in Thousand Oaks to saying, "Okay, we better get serious about how you roll out this drug in France. What is it about those healthcare systems that's unique?" . . . We have to be prepared internally when new data comes in so that we can very quickly move to the next stage. We were fully geared up to move to whatever that next stage was.

Within days of the global summit in Rome, Amgen received the results of the phase II trial. The results were surprising—and extremely deflating. The phase II trial had fallen short of its endpoint of improving patients' motor scores by 25 percent. The trial had failed.

Patients on GDNF improved by 10 percent and those on placebo by 4.5 percent, but there were too few patients to conclude that the 5.5 percent difference between the two groups was statistically significant. The PET scans of the patients on GDNF showed an increase in dopamine storage in the brain, but those physiological changes apparently had not translated into a real-life improvement in motor function. It was devastating news, and it meant the company would have to rethink its plans for a phase III trial.[28]

Amgen officials called their counterparts at Medtronic in late June and gave them the disappointing report. On June 28, 2004, Amgen issued a press release about the failed phase II trial:

> Amgen, the world's largest biotechnology company, today announced that the Phase 2 study of its novel glial cell line-derived neurotrophic factor, or GDNF, for the treatment of

> advanced Parkinson's disease did not meet the primary study endpoint upon completion of six months of the double-blind treatment phase of the study. In the study, GDNF was safe and well-tolerated. . . .
>
> We are currently analyzing the data to understand why this study differs from the long-term improvement of the patients, who have been treated with GDNF for close to three years in an ongoing open-label study being conducted in the United Kingdom," said Beth Seidenberg, M.D., chief medical officer and senior vice president, Amgen. "We are committed to understanding if a different approach, including evaluating a higher dose, may yield an outcome that is consistent with the open label study.[29]

When it became clear that GDNF wouldn't be launched commercially any time soon, Amgen assigned Michael Reilly to the GDNF project. He had joined Amgen in 1998 and, by July of 2004, was the company's director of global marketing. He specialized in helping to design clinical trials that would lead to commercial development. The question now was whether the company should make a second attempt at a phase II trial or abandon the pump-and-catheter delivery method altogether.

Amgen organized a meeting with the principal investigators of the failed phase II trial. The group discussed possible reasons the trial had failed. Dr. Gill from Bristol suggested that the difference in catheter size might be to blame. It was possible that the patients in the phase II trial weren't getting the drug because it was refluxing up the catheter track. Dr. Hutchinson from NYU submitted that the statistical analysis of the phase II data might have been flawed; perhaps there were subgroups of patients (younger patients, patients with less-advanced forms of the disease) that responded better to GDNF than most. The majority view, though, was that the dose of the phase II trial was simply too low to be effective. The patients had been given 15 µg a day on each side of the brain. The average dose in the original Bristol trial had been 25 µg a day and the daily dose in Kentucky was 30 µg. At least one of the investigators suggested increasing the dose to as high as 45 µg a day, but the majority settled on 30 µg a day as dose that would be safe and hopefully effective.

The company decided to conduct another phase II trial. According to Mr. Reilly, this was done on the strength of the earlier animal trials and the phase I trials in Bristol and Kentucky. He said, "[The reasoning] was, 'Hey it looks pretty safe. We continue to see long-term results in these uncontrolled trials. Why don't we give one last effort?' . . . We decided to do it one last time, once again, on the back of the clinical and preclinical trials."

At this point Amgen had spent at least $400 million invested in GDNF, including the acquisition of Synergen in 1994 and more than $150 million spent in animal and clinical trials during the intervening decade. Mr. Reilly said Amgen was unusually committed to GDNF, probably because of how promising it seemed in early trials. "That's more effort than Amgen usually puts in to develop a drug," he said.

Throughout July of 2004, Mr. Reilly, Dr. Masterman, and others began to write the protocol for the new phase II trial. If the results of that trial were stark enough—if the higher dose brought about the same results seen in Bristol and Kentucky—it was possible that the FDA could approve the GDNF for market straight away. If not, Amgen would probably have to conduct a full-fledged phase III trial, which would add on at least another six months of development time.

If the death of Mickey Traub and the negative results of the phase II trial were the first and second strikes against GDNF, the third and fourth strikes came almost simultaneously in August of 2004.

Antibodies

By the summer of 2004, Amgen's scientists knew that one patient had developed antibodies to the manmade GDNF. Antibodies are proteins that the immune system dispatches to deal with unfamiliar substances, and in this patient's case, the antibodies had begun to latch onto and neutralize the man-made GDNF. Amgen's scientist feared that the antibodies might also neutralize the GDNF that occurs naturally in the human body. It is known that GDNF plays an important role in the brain of a developing fetus, but it isn't clear what naturally occurring GDNF does, if anything, for the adult brain. If the patient's antibodies began to attack the natural GDNF, bad things might happen or nothing might happen. Fortunately, the patient with the antibodies hadn't reported any negative side effects, but Amgen was watching closely. After discovering antibodies in that one patient, Amgen had ordered that each of the four dozen or so patients still on GDNF be tested for the antibodies.

In mid-August of 2004, those test results came back. Amgen learned that two more patients in the phase II trial and one patient from the original Bristol trial had developed antibodies. One patient had reported some upper-body muscle weakness, but it wasn't clear whether this was related to the antibodies.

Toxicology

The fourth strike, and the one that was universally acknowledged to be the most fatal to the trials, came on the heels of the third. Amgen learned in August of 2004 that two monkeys on GDNF had suffered irreversible brain damage.

While the phase II trial was going on, Amgen also had been testing GDNF in a group of monkeys to satisfy the FDA's requirements for animal toxicology studies. The company had contracted with a research laboratory called Northern Biomedical Research Inc. in Michigan to pump GDNF into the brains of the monkeys at varying doses. The 59 monkeys were divided into four groups: a control group that got none of the drug and groups that received either 15, 30, or 100 µg a day. The purpose of the study was to determine whether GDNF would become toxic and destroy brain tissue at high doses.

Fifteen of the monkeys were put in the "high-dose group" and got GDNF at a rate of 100 µg a day, a higher dose than any human had received. Most of them, ten of the 15, got the drug for six months and then were euthanized, their bodies frozen. The other five monkeys in the high-dose group received GDNF for six months and then had the drug abruptly withdrawn and replaced with saline solution for a three-month "recovery" period.

A veteran veterinary pathologist named Mark T. Butt at Charles River Laboratories Inc. in Maryland performed the necropsy and examined their brains at the microscopic level. What he discovered, he immediately reported to his contact at Amgen: two of the monkeys in the high-dose group had strange and severe lesions on the cerebellum.

Both monkeys were part of the minority that received GDNF for six months and then received the saline placebo for another three months. Dr. Butt later stated that he called his contact at Amgen immediately: "Because the cerebellar findings were so unique and unexpected, and because I was aware that GDNF clinical trials with human subjects were ongoing, I immediately . . . telephoned the study monitor at Amgen."[30]

The news could not have come at a worse time. With the death of Dr. Traub, the dismal phase II trial results, the new cases of antibodies, and now the brain-damaged monkeys, fate seemed to be conspiring against the GDNF trials. In addition, Amgen had just begun to draw up plans for a new trial that would *increase* the dose of GDNF. Could the company justify a higher dose in the face of such sobering toxicology results?

Dr. Roger Perlmutter had been involved with the GDNF trials since joining Amgen in 2001. Though Mr. Reilly was not personally a part of the group that made the final decision to halt the trials, he said Drs. Roger Perlmutter and Donna Masterman would have been.

"I can't say who all was in the room when that happened, but I can guarantee you that Donna and Roger were part of the group that was looking at it," Mr. Riley said. "We're a publicly traded company, and these types of things we have to keep fairly close because they're material, and so you need the right people in the room; but they don't invite extras, even someone like me that's pretty close."

In a statement he made many months later, Dr. Perlmutter described how Amgen went about deciding the future of the GDNF trials:

> Amgen employed a risk-benefit analysis in determining whether to halt the phase II studies. The benefit factor was zero, because the unblinding of the study revealed no efficacy of GDNF as compared to placebo. Any risk, weighed against a lack of any benefit at all, would weigh in favor of not continuing the study. In this case, the risks were grave.[31]

On September 1, 2004, Amgen's GDNF project leaders called the lead investigators at the trial sites around the world. Every GDNF trial—the phase I trials in Bristol and Kentucky and the phase II trial—was to be halted immediately. The pumps were to be drained of GDNF, rinsed, and switched off. The investigators were to notify their patients as soon as possible.

Amgen also sent a letter by fax that outlined the company's reasons for halting the trials. The letter described the puzzling toxicology data ("The exact cause of the lesions is unknown thus far, but these observation warrant considerable concern."), and the new instances of antibodies. It was signed by Dr. Masterman, Amgen's associate director of medical sciences, and it concluded this way:

> Amgen is deeply saddened by the need to discontinue the [GDNF] program. We recognize that the Parkinson's community desperately needs safe and effective therapeutics to treat the disease, and we had all hoped that [GDNF] would prove to be a breakthrough in the treatment of PD.

19 A Dark Day

Roger and Linda Thacker had been anxious to meet their fellow GDNF volunteers for almost a year. Dr. Slevin and the others at Kentucky had asked them not to communicate with the other patients during the trial to avoid skewing the results. They didn't want to compromise the study, and so they complied; but now that the formal study was over, the Thackers were excited to share their success stories and hear those of the other patients. They asked if the doctors might arrange a meeting of the trial volunteers. To accommodate the Thackers' request and similar requests from other patients, the Kentucky doctors organized a dinner party. It was scheduled for a Wednesday in the fall of 2004—on September 1.

The party took place at the Stanley Demos' Coach House restaurant in downtown Lexington. Roger said he knew something was wrong soon after he arrived. "There was no one from Amgen there," he said. Amgen's Dr. Masterman was supposed to have attended along with other Amgen employees. The doctors and nurses at the party seemed a little on edge. Roger tried to enjoy the party. He mingled with the other patients and swapped stories with them about what the drug had done for him. Every Kentucky patient had chosen to continue receiving GDNF after the study, which meant every patient who attended the party was carrying a pump in the abdomen and a catheter in the brain.

Dr. Slevin was present, but he wasn't enjoying the party. He had received a phone call earlier that day from Amgen telling him to take GDNF away from his patients. He had told the other Kentucky doctors the bad news. The party had been planned for weeks, and the doctors decided to allow it to go ahead as planned.

"We decided to keep it quiet. We didn't want to ruin the party," he said later. He called the patients the following day.

* * *

September 1, 2004, was a dark day for the GDNF patients. On that date or shortly thereafter, each received word that the trials were over. Some of the principal investigators contacted their patients directly by phone, some delegated the dreadful task to a nurse or a co-investigator, and some let their patients know in person. Before the trials were cut short, 48 patients were receiving GDNF in Bristol, Kentucky, Virginia, Toronto, Chicago, New York, North Carolina, and Oregon.

Amgen had not consulted with the study doctors before halting the trials, and the company's decision came to them as a shock. They exchanged e-mails in the days following the decision and discussed the ethics of taking GDNF away. They contacted the company about their concerns. The e-mails indicate that most of the investigators initially expressed some degree of concern that Amgen's decision was unethical.

Steve Gill, the neurosurgeon from Bristol who had organized the first successful trial of GDNF, sent a letter to Donna Masterman, co-leader of Amgen's GDNF team. He wrote it two days after

Amgen ended the trials. It reflects the dismay of both the patients and the investigators:

> I am sure you will be aware that Amgen's decision to halt all clinical dosing of [GDNF] has had a devastating impact on all the patients who agreed to participate in the various trials. Individuals in our phase I study have now been treated with [GDNF] for three and half years, all remain well and are leading full and independent lives which prior to treatment was not at all possible. Prior to treatment their prospects were of progressive decline from a state of severe incapacity. All of my patients without exception have been very distressed by this news and have asked me to contact you on their behalf requesting that Amgen reconsider their decision. My personal view is that Amgen's decision to halt the clinical trials is premature and there should at least have been the opportunity for the clinical investigators to discuss the new findings before we received a directive from you.

Dr. Gill went on to question the company's reasons for stopping the trials—the brain damage to the monkeys and the presence of neutralizing antibodies. He wrote that not only were the monkeys receiving far higher doses than any human ever had, but the nature of the brain damage suggested that it was caused by something other than GDNF. The antibodies were indeed a concern and should be watched closely, he wrote, but similar antibodies had not kept other treatments from being developed and coming to market.

In closing, he wrote, "I wonder if there is still time to take further advice and reconsider the wisdom of this precipitate decision which is likely to come under intense scrutiny by patient groups and the scientific community."

Amgen had apparently not responded to Dr. Gill's concerns one week later because at that point Anthony Lang, a veteran neurologist who was lead investigator at the site in Toronto, wrote in an e-mail to the other investigators, "I have also been pushing Donna [Masterman to] formally respond to the concerns raised by Steve [Gill]. So far, the silence is deafening."

Some of the investigators found themselves deeply conflicted. They had seen their patients improve on GDNF, but now Amgen had given specific instructions to withdraw the drug. By taking it away without good reason, wouldn't they violate the principal tenet of the Hippocratic Oath to "first do no harm?"

To take a stand against Amgen might mean jeopardizing future research grants and other perks that went along with working in conjunction with a cash-laden drug company—the five-star dinners, the summits in exotic locations.

Dr. Slevin said his contacts at Amgen were anxious to have the pumps turned off and taken out quickly. "They wanted it all out and done and over with—and then obviously it's not a headache for them. It's done, it's gone, there's no recourse." But he and his colleagues at Kentucky did not immediately comply.

"We talked about it and we ran through what happens when you stop [the pump] then start it again. The other thing was, what happens if cooler heads prevailed after a week or two, or a month or so, and we decided we'll restart it? . . . I think the primary idea was that nobody's going to be hurt by getting one more day of this stuff or a week or two. The idea was that we didn't precipitously change things. We put it off two to three weeks. . . . That gave us more time to consolidate our thoughts."

Dr. Hutchinson at NYU refused to withdraw the drug until the toxicology data was better understood. He did so after conferring with NYU's Ethics Committee and with the Internal Review Board, both of which gave him permission to keep providing the drug. He continued to give GDNF to his patients until the quantities he had on hand were spent.

Not all of the investigators were so conflicted. Jay Nutt, the lead investigator for the Oregon site, wrote in response to an e-mail from Dr. Gill that he had not seen his patients improve: "After talking to Donna Masterman it was clear that Amgen is not going forward with the trial. . . . As none of our patients had improved with GDNF, there was no ethical issue in stopping the pumps. We have reluctantly done so."

Dr. Tony Lang in Toronto, Dr. Mark Stacy at Duke, and Dr. Frederick Wooten at UVA likewise had their patients' pumps shut off. They later said they had not seen a significant improvement in their patients.

Dr. Gill's prediction that Amgen would come under intense scrutiny by the patient and research communities proved to be prescient. In the weeks and months that followed, patients and investigators involved in the trials became more public in their criticisms. The hottest debate centered on the damaged brains of two monkeys.

20 Withdrawal Phenomenon

Despite the other strikes against them, clinical trials of GDNF would likely have continued were it not for brain damage discovered in the two monkeys, according to former Amgen employees and lead investigators. The other complications were worrisome, they say, but the brain damage was the deal-breaker.

Michael Reilly, who co-led the GDNF team, said, "I think the antibody issue would have resulted in additional safety precautions being added to the trial and additional monitoring and perhaps additional understanding to what was causing that," he said. "The toxicology I think was more worrisome than the antibodies. The antibody issue was like, you don't like to see it [and] you don't understand it. But on the other hand we're not a company that sees bad toxicology results, bad potentially certain side effect results, and then waits to see bad results in man."

Dr. Hutchinson, the lead investigator at NYU, said that during a phone call with Roger Perlmutter, Amgen's VP of research and development, Perlmutter said the antibodies were not a major concern: "I said, 'What are you going to do about the lesions and neutralizing antibodies?' He said he wasn't at all worried about the antibodies. It just meant these antibodies bind to the drug and make it less effective. That's why he wasn't worried about it."

The sudden death of Dr. Traub, the failed phase II trial, and the antibodies all were roadblocks, but it was the lesioned brains of two monkeys that undid the GDNF trials. Naturally these monkeys became a focal point of debate. No one questioned whether the brain damage had occurred, but there began to be serious disagreement about what caused it. Amgen's scientists believed GDNF itself was to blame, so they had ordered the trials to be halted abruptly.

Dr. Hutchinson suggested an alternative explanation. He was on vacation in England when Amgen announced the end of the trials and didn't see the toxicology report for more than a week. When he did finally see the report, he noticed something odd about the data.

In total, 15 monkeys had received the highest dose of GDNF. All 15 had the drug pumped into their brain at the same rate. Ten of the 15 had received the high dose for six months and were euthanized. The other five received the high dose for six months, had it abruptly withdrawn at six months and then were kept alive for three months before being euthanized. Both monkeys that were found to have brain damage had been part of this smaller group—the group from whom GDNF had been abruptly withdrawn. To Dr. Hutchinson, it sounded a lot like withdrawal phenomenon.

Withdrawal phenomenon occurs when cells become saturated with a protein, such as GDNF, and then implode when the protein is abruptly taken away. The cells grow accustomed to the protein-rich environment; and when that environment suddenly changes, their walls collapse and they die. It's not the protein itself that causes the brain damage but rather the abrupt withdrawal of the protein.

Dr. Hutchinson suggested that the abrupt withdrawal of GDNF might have caused the brain damage. It was possible that at such a high dose, the cerebella of the monkeys had become so saturated in GDNF that when it was withdrawn at six months, the cells collapsed and brain damage ensued.

Whether or not Hutchinson was right, Amgen had a clear incentive to reject his hypothesis. If abrupt withdrawal *had* caused the lesions, the company would appear at best foolish and at worst reckless for not having considered the possibility before unilaterally halting the trials. And if abrupt withdrawal of GDNF had caused irreversible brain damage in monkeys, the last thing the company should have done would be to order the *abrupt withdrawal* from human patients, which is precisely what Amgen did.

The investigators who followed Amgen's instructions, and turned off their patients' pumps without protest, also would risk looking foolish or irresponsible. Shouldn't they have considered the risks of withdrawal phenomenon before heeding Amgen's instruction to shut off the pumps? The research community may be critical of such easy compliance. They, too, had a clear incentive to reject the withdrawal phenomenon explanation.

Controversial as it was, to Dr. Hutchinson it was the most logical explanation of why brain damage would occur only among the five monkeys that had been abruptly withdrawn and not in the other 10.

"It just took me 20 minutes to figure it out. What do these animals have in common? They were all quickly withdrawn," he said. "I called Roger Perlmutter. He called back September ninth and said he hadn't thought of that."

Amgen did not immediately respond to Dr. Hutchinson's concerns. By the time he raised them, several GDNF patients, including those in Oregon, already had been taken off the drug—abruptly. The implications of withdrawal phenomenon were enormous. If it were true, it would undermine Amgen's core reason for halting the trial. It would also mean that the patients who already had been taken off the drug had been exposed to the very risk Amgen was attempting to avoid: the possibility of brain damage.

21 The Fourth Monkey

A new discovery several weeks after the trials ended seemed to settle the matter. Amgen had reexamined the 59 monkeys from the toxicology study and discovered two additional monkeys with similar lesions on their brains. One of these monkeys, like the original two, had received GDNF for six months and then had it abruptly taken away. These three lent credibility to Dr. Hutchinson's explanation of withdrawal phenomenon.

But there was a fourth monkey. That monkey had also received the high dose for six months, but instead of being kept alive for another three months without GDNF, the monkey was immediately euthanized at six months, with no recovery period. The monkey had received the high dose but hadn't experienced the abrupt withdrawal, yet the animal had suffered similar brain damage. The fourth monkey cast serious doubt on Hutchinson's explanation. If withdrawal were to blame, why would a monkey that received GDNF until the time of its death suffer brain damage?

Amgen organized a quasi-independent group of pathologists to examine the data. The Pathology Working Group, or PWG, included two Amgen doctors, two from companies with whom Amgen had contracted to conduct the toxicology study in the monkeys, a pathologist from Stanford University named Linda Cork, and a veterinary pathology consultant named Robert Garman. According to a sworn affidavit by Mark T. Butt, the pathologist who discovered the lesions in the first place and who was a member of the six-person group, the PWG rejected the withdrawal phenomenon hypothesis because of that fourth monkey:

> The PWG . . . considered whether withdrawal of GDNF might have played a role in causing the cerebellar damage observed in the three primates from the high dose recovery group. The PWG concluded that this was unlikely since the same lesions observed in the primates from the high dose recovery group were present, albeit in a milder form, in the cerebellum of one of the primates from the high dose treatment group. Based upon the PWG's interpretation of the cerebellar lesions, the panel concluded that there was no value in tapering versus immediately discontinuing GDNF treatment.[32]

The group concluded that there was unlikely to be any risk in withdrawing patients abruptly. The investigators who continued to provide GDNF, contrary to Amgen's wishes, knew that eventually they would have no choice but to withdraw the drug. They had only limited quantities of GDNF on hand; and because Amgen stopped providing the drug, they would have to substitute saline solution for the drug when GDNF ran out. By late October, each of the investigators—some grudgingly, some willingly—had taken GDNF from their patients.

22 Publicity

Kristen Suthers, the youngest of Bob's and Elaine's three daughters, was doing post-doctorate work at Johns Hopkins University in Baltimore when her father joined the GDNF study. After Bob's stroke, Kristen and her sisters visited him in the hospital. They had seen Parkinson's and a heart condition assail their father physically, but his active mind had remained intact. Kristen said that to see him after the stroke was overwhelming. "I just remember so well my sister right after the stroke saying, 'The one thing he had left was his mind.'"

Kristen hadn't wanted her father to continue in the study but supported his decision to do so. She had seen him give a lot to the GDNF trials, and now Amgen was taking the drug away. Kristen had earned a master's degree in public health at NYU and a PhD. in gerontology from the University of Southern California. After learning about Amgen's reasons for halting the trial, she thought it was all just a misunderstanding, a miscalculation. On one hand, she believed that Amgen had undervalued the drug's positive effects in the phase II patients. On the other, the company had reacted too hastily to the toxicology results in the monkey trial. If she could show the company what the drug had done for the patients, of course Amgen would reconsider.

Two months after the trials ended she started a Web site called GDNF4Parkinsons.org and on it posted testimonials from patients involved in the GDNF study. Amgen's scientists would read it, realize their mistake and resume the trials.

"I just figured, I'm going to make a Web site. I'm going to tell everyone's story. I was so naïve at that point. I thought the company just didn't know what was going on, and if I could show Amgen what GDNF had done for these people, Amgen would do the right thing. . . . We just kept thinking, the company is going to do the right thing."

Meanwhile, in Chicago, Maggie Kaufman had been building up a network of GDNF patients, family members, and friends. She first sent e-mails to the Kentucky doctors and to Dr. Gill in Bristol. She introduced herself as the wife of Steve Kaufman, a GDNF patient, and asked the doctors to pass her contact information on to their patients. By mid-September, patients at both sites had contacted her by phone or e-mail. The network expanded to include friends and distant relatives, acquaintances with some knowledge of the FDA, the pharmaceutical industry or the like. Maggie made contact with Roger and Linda Thacker in Kentucky and with another Kentucky patient named Eddie Abney, who became and remained actively involved in the effort.

Steve Kaufman wrote a letter to the Michael J. Fox Foundation on September 30, 2004. He described his improvements on GDNF and asked if the foundation would use its mighty influence to help the patients recover the drug. Around the same time, Maggie Kaufman called every major Parkinson's research organization in the United States. All the major players said there was nothing they could do to help. She discovered that the organizations were well-equipped to raise money for Parkinson's research or to lobby the government, but they had no real mechanism for challenging the decision of a large, privately held company. She found a sympathetic ear at the New York-based Parkinson's Disease Foundation and the D.C.-based Parkinson's Action Network. Both groups eventually made formal declarations of support for the patients, urging Amgen to reconsider.

In October, Andrew Pollack, a reporter for the *New York Times* who writes about biotechnology, called Steve Kaufman and asked for an interview. To the Kaufman's, his call was a sign that their fight was gaining traction.

Another sign came when the Kaufmans received a call from the Fox Foundation. The question of whether Amgen had erred in ending the trials was becoming highly divisive in the Parkinson's community. Rather than take sides, the Fox Foundation instead teamed with the Kinetics Foundation to organize a meeting of experienced scientists to examine Amgen's decision. The two foundations had organized a similar summit in 2003 to discuss the lackluster trial results of some controversial fetal tissue transplant trials. That the foundation would go to such lengths to discuss GDNF reflects the high profile GDNF had achieved in the Parkinson's community and the expectations of it before it was pulled. The meeting would take place in mid-November 2004.

Around the same time the Fox summit took place, Maggie Kaufman combined efforts with Kristen Suthers, and the two women remained at the center of the patients' coordinated effort to recover GDNF. Kristen had begun posting patient testimonials on her Web site, and Maggie used her network of contacts to invite other patients to share their experiences.

23 GDNF Summit

The GDNF summit took place in New York City during two days in late October of 2004, and it involved some 30 scientists and representatives from patient organizations. Most of the lead investigators from the three GDNF trials were present. Dr. Lang, the principal investigator for the phase II site in Toronto, co-chaired the meeting with William Langston, the director of the Parkinson's Institute in Sunnyvale, California and the chief scientific adviser to the Fox Foundation. Donna Masterman and Michael Reilly from Amgen were present, as was a representative from Medtronic. (Five of the scientists, none of whom were lead investigators for the GDNF trials, later wrote a summary of the discussion titled "Crossroads in GDNF Therapy for Parkinson's Disease" that was published in the journal *Movement Disorders* in early 2006 —more than one year after the summit itself.)[33]

In the meeting the scientists attempted to reconcile the different outcomes of the phase I and phase II trials. They also evaluated the two main safety issues of the phase II trial: the GDNF antibodies and the brain damage in the monkeys.

The published report on the summit describes the challenges in drawing any conclusions about the trials. For example, each trial used a different type of catheter and each used different dosing levels. The Bristol and Kentucky trials relied on convection-enhanced delivery (GDNF driven into the tissue under pressure), but the phase II trial did not. Of the three types used, the summit report identifies Dr. Gill's invention as the most effective: "Of all the studies, the catheter used in the Bristol study appears to have had the best design to promote the convection-enhanced delivery of GDNF, as the path of least resistance was out the single hole and most likely into surrounding tissue and not back up the catheter track."[34]

The Kentucky catheter was larger than the one used in Bristol and more likely to create a channel around the catheter, but it also had 40 holes along its tip and achieved the "soaker hose" effect. The catheter used in the phase II study, however, was a step backward even from the Kentucky catheter: it did not allow convection-enhanced delivery, and it had only a single hole in its tip, making it the most likely of the three to shoot the drug back along the catheter track instead of into the tissue of the putamen. Yet the authors of the report are reluctant to conclude that the catheters alone explain the different results in the phase I and phase II trials.

> Without an accurate way of measuring GDNF diffusion in living patients, uncertainty remains as to whether the differences in efficacy across these studies can be partially explained by differences in the catheters and GDNF bioavailability," the report stated. "Currently there has been no systematic study to compare the effectiveness of each of the catheters and infusion rates used to deliver GDNF, and for this reason, a systematic study to compare catheter systems in [monkeys] appears to be warranted.[35]

In other words, the best way to know which catheter and dose are most effective is to carry out an animal study that directly compares the three catheter types at various doses. "These studies will have implications beyond GDNF therapy. . . ," states the report.

The doctors also discussed placebo effect. "Both the Bristol and the Kentucky trials were conducted in an open-label fashion with both the patient and physicians aware of GDNF delivery. The double-blind study was conducted so that neither the patients nor the physicians knew whether the patient received GDNF or [placebo]. A simple explanation for the different clinical results, and the reason controlled trials are so critical, is the placebo effect. Previous studies have shown that PD patients are especially sensitive to placebo effects, which may be sustained for prolonged periods of time, particularly in response to invasive surgical procedures."[36]

The report then refers to several studies in which the placebo effect was surprisingly strong. In one famous study, Parkinson's patients had tissue from pig fetuses implanted in their brains. After 18 months, those who had received the fetal tissue had improved by 25 percent. Patients in the same study who underwent a fake surgery and received no new tissue, improved by 22 percent. Other studies showed real, physiological changes in Parkinson's patients on placebo, suggesting the effects weren't simply imagined but actual, physical results of anticipating treatment. Placebo effect, in other words, could account for some of the improvements in some of the GDNF patients.

But the report then points to the original Bristol trial as evidence that there's more to GDNF than placebo effect. Those five patients, including Henry Webb, Stephen Waite and Richard Hembrough, received GDNF almost continuously for more than three years.

"The open-label trial from Bristol suggested that not all the benefit could be explained by placebo effect. This evidence included progressive improvement in clinical benefit that was sustained for more than 3 years [and] failure of that benefit to decline after GDNF withdrawal. . . ."[37] In effect, the report states that either GDNF was curing those patients in England or the Bristol trial is possibly the most extreme example of placebo effect in the history of Parkinson's treatment.

The report offers little new about the neutralizing antibodies discovered in about 10 percent of the GDNF patients. It encourages more research to determine whether the antibodies affected the body's naturally occurring GDNF or just the synthetic version of the protein. The report also advises that the GDNF patients be monitored long term to see if any negative effects arise. "The lack of any obvious negative effects in those patients with such antibodies over time would be reassuring," the report states.[38]

When the conversation at the meeting turned to the brain damage in the monkeys, Dr. Hutchinson was well prepared. He had invited Kim Heidenreich, a pharmacologist and professor at the University of Colorado at Denver Health Sciences Center. One of Dr. Heidenreich's research interests is the cell death that occurs when a protein is abruptly withdrawn from the brain. She had been involved in a study that showed that withdrawal phenomenon could cause the same type of brain damage seen in the GDNF-treated monkeys.[39] Dr. Hutchinson invited her to the summit so that she could give her assessment of the brain damage in the monkeys. She said on that day (and repeated to me in an interview nearly two years later) that she believes the brain damage in the GDNF monkeys is consistent with withdrawal phenomenon. "I definitely believe it was withdrawal phenomenon," she told me during the telephone interview.

The published report makes no mention of Dr. Heidenreich, but it does acknowledge withdrawal phenomenon as a possible—though remote—explanation of the brain damage: "It is possible that GDNF withdrawal contributed to the cerebellar toxicity. . . . However, the finding of similar pathology in an animal that was not withdrawn from GDNF casts doubt on this hypothesis."[40]

Once again, scientists pointed to the fourth monkey as evidence that withdrawal phenomenon couldn't have caused the brain damage. The report ends with a section titled, "Where do we go from here?" The answer to that question, the doctors write, is that the research community needs to resolve the safety issues before GDNF can be pumped into the human brain again. The report urges that future GDNF trials be carefully designed to produce conclusive results, a not-so-subtle criticism of the design of the inconclusive phase II trial.

24 Letter Campaign

The Fox summit came and went with no change in the patients' status. Throughout October and November 2004 the patients and their families wrote letters and sent e-mails to Amgen employees. This letter, included here in its entirety, was sent by Linda Thacker, the wife of Kentucky patient Roger Thacker. It is representative in content and tone of dozens of others sent during that period.

To: **Amgen**
Ms. Donna Masterman
Amgen Inc.
1 Amgen Center Drive
Thousand Oaks, California 91320-1799

Please allow me to introduce myself. My name is Linda Thacker. I am the wife of Roger Thacker or, as he is known in the GDNF research study at the University of Kentucky, [patient No.]107.

I am writing to you because you have stopped the study, broken our contract to receive the GDNF for two years and we are told the possibility of your changing your mind is slim to none.

I woke up this morning thinking about our situation. This is not surprising since I toss and turn all night struggling to understand what has happened to us.

Before Parkinson's disease, my husband's life and living since birth has been involved with animals. Livestock, wildlife, zoological research; you name it he has handled it. Roger owns/operates a once-active farming operation. He also supplied and transported livestock southeast region wide. In addition to this he has held the position of Chair of the Natural Resource Council for the American Sheep Industry, specializing in such areas as endangered species, land management, and water availability. Holding such a position entailed a certain amount of travel nationwide, which we both enjoyed. Roger also provided pertinent background data for several individual senators in the United States congress who are active in the natural resource area.

Roger has had Parkinson's disease for at least eight years. Before Dr. Slevin introduced him to GDNF his decline was slow but steady. Upon entering the GDNF program Roger lived with constant pain and rigidity in his body. This affected his ability to balance, walk, talk, sit alone, feed, bath, or dress himself. He was seldom able to leave his home or socialize with friends and family. Roger was unable to sleep for more than an hour before needing to be moved to relieve the pain and rigidity in his body (day and night). This took a great toll on his health and that of his primary caregiver, me.

After being on GDNF for just a few weeks the pain subsided. Gradually his ability to move, balance and care for his personal needs independently increased. He began to work on his farm. His ability to drive returned enough that he drove himself around the farm to do chores. He began to return to the activities of the family and as husband and wife we laughed together again.

Since the removal of the GDNF my husband's decline again is steady. Again, pain is his constant companion and our lives again are on survival mode. Roger is slipping away from us and we want to know why? What justification can you give us for condemning him and our family in this manner?

Ten people in Kentucky were invited into this study. Ten people who were suffering with a disease so horrible that they felt it a gift to be offered a chance to put their lives on the line to help find better treatments for Parkinson's Disease.

It was hard at times, it was demanding of both the research team and the patients. But we all did it—everything that was asked of us. Because the research team is a group of scientists and doctors of complete honesty, integrity and compassion. And the patients, each one of them, are fine, intelligent, brave individuals from all walks of life. They are fathers, mothers, sons, and daughters. They are people who are suffering and they do not deserve to. They are our loved ones. They are important!

When I awoke this morning I felt impressed to go to my dictionary. I turned to the word "coward." It read, "A person who lacks courage." I then looked up the word "courage." Webster defines it as, "The quality of being brave." I then turned to the word "brave." It is defined as "not afraid, having courage."

I then understood what it is that I want to know. What is it you are afraid of? You have never come to meet us. You have not heard our stories. You have not studied the two years of our research, before and after GDNF. It is available, both in data and videotapes.

GDFN does work! It stopped my husband's pain, it gave him quality on time (mobility). He is a husband who could hug his wife again. Once again this has been taken from me. He is a father who was not able to participate in the four years of his honor student daughter's high school experience. With GDNF we were planning to visit her college campus in Boulder, Colorado. Our grandchildren can no longer play spontaneously with their grandpa. This is cheating these little ones of all the wonderful things grandpa can teach them. The families of each of the participants in the Kentucky program have their own stories of hope and life regained, only to have it snatched from them. Your decision has been devastating for us.

What are you afraid of? Come face us, sit down with us and tell us how allowing us to continue receiving GDNF as we were promised can be such a threat. I know if you will meet with us, we could come to an agreement that would calm your fears and allow compassionate use to be successfully put in place. These brave individuals and their families deserve this. Time and immediate action is so critical. The pumps, tubes and shunts are in place. Nothing you fear in giving these courageous people back the GDNF can possibly match the fear we feel in facing the future without it.

This is what it comes to. We are at your mercy. You hold the cards to the quality of life that our families will experience from here on out. Won't you reconsider? My husband and I will not be able to sleep well at night (not by choice but due to pain and rigidity) until the GDNF is restored. What I ask is how can you sleep at night knowing that you have not done all you can to know and understand the success of the GDNF research study at the University of Kentucky and the devastating impact your decision has had on so many lives.

Sincerely,
Linda Thacker

25 A Second Chance

Within a few weeks of the Fox Foundation summit on GDNF, Amgen flew the principal investigators to its headquarters in Thousand Oaks. Other investigators, including Don Gash from Kentucky, also were present. Dr. Gash said it was at that meeting that the polarization of the investigators became apparent. The eight lead investigators split more or less evenly down the middle. Four supported the company's decision to stop the trials. These were Dr. Lang from Toronto, Dr. Nutt from Oregon, Dr. Stacy from Duke, and Dr. Wooten from the University of Virginia. These four attributed much of the patients' perceived improvements to the placebo effect, and they agreed with Amgen that the safety issues were too great to continue the trials.

The other four remained critical of the company's decision. These four said they had seen their patient improve noticeably on GDNF, and they were skeptical about Amgen's reasons for halting the trials. These four were Dr. Gill in Bristol, Dr. Hutchinson at NYU, Dr. Penn in Chicago, and Dr. Slevin in Kentucky. At the meeting in mid-November in Thousand Oaks, Dr. Gash later said, it became obvious there was a "polarization within the groups of investigators."

During the meeting, Dr. Gash inquired about a letter that the University of Kentucky had sent to Amgen in early September. In the letter, the university had offered to take over the trial and assume liability for the nine Kentucky patients. He asked whether Amgen would be willing to consent to the arrangement. According to Dr. Gash, Amgen's Donna Masterman said no, and Dr. Penn from Chicago asked why not. Dr. Gash later said that "Donna Masterman got up and presented the FDA guidelines and said there's no way the FDA would allow us to go ahead with the drug." At that point Dr. Penn asked if Amgen would be willing to meet with the FDA to discuss the possibility of the universities taking over as sponsors of the trials. In theory, the arrangement would free Amgen from liability and allow the trials to continue.

"They [Amgen] said they would," Dr. Gash recalled. "I think they were confident the FDA was going to turn us down."

Dr. Penn, who had consulted for the FDA for years, believed the federal agency might allow the trials to resume, provided he and the other investigators could make a convincing case that GDNF was safe and effective.

Amgen formally requested a meeting with the FDA's Center for Drug Evaluation and Research, and the date was set in early January of 2005. The company made clear that it would act as a facilitator in the meeting but that the discussion would mainly involve the FDA and the principal investigators.

26 Change of Momentum

Elaine Suthers began writing letters almost immediately after the trials ended. She wrote to each of Amgen's board of directors, to CEO Kevin Sharer, and VP of Research Roger Perlmutter. She wrote to her friends and asked that they do the same. Usually the letters went unanswered. If an answer did come it arrived as a form letter printed on Amgen's letterhead or as a boilerplate e-mail. The weeks passed and Thanksgiving came. The Suthers celebrated the holiday in their Long Island home with their children and grandchildren. The GDNF controversy dominated the conversation at the dinner table.

Then, on the morning after Thanksgiving day, 2004, the patients' story beat out the countless other disasters and scandals that compete each day for the front page of the *New York Times*. Andrew Pollack's article appeared under the headline, "Many See Hope in Parkinson's Drug Pulled from Testing" and began with a description of Steve Kaufman from Chicago.

The article triggered an avalanche of media coverage of the GDNF patients. Diane Sawyer, front woman of ABC's *Good Morn-*

ing America, read the *Times* article and immediately decided to put the GDNF patients on the show. A *GMA* producer called the Kaufmans on the same day that the story ran on the front page of the *Times*. Maggie Kaufman put the producer in touch with the Thackers, who as Long Island residents were much closer to *GMA*'s studio in New York City. ABC sent news crews to Chicago to interview the Kaufmans and to Kentucky to interview several patients there. Local news agencies followed suit. The *Lexington Herald-Leader* published a lengthy front-page article just before Christmas.

Encouraged by the new national attention, Bob and Elaine sent letters to Amgen executives and to the company's board of directors. They wrote to their local representatives in congress and asked their friends to do the same. By Christmas of 2004 the Suthers, the Kaufmans, and the other patients were feeling a surge of momentum behind their cause, pushing them into the spotlight. They knew Amgen would be feeling the pressure.

The *Good Morning America* report aired December 28. It began with a pre-recorded interview of Barbara Allen, a school teacher from the Lexington area who was one of the 10 GDNF patients there. The report included dramatic before-and-after footage of Ms. Allen as she completed a basic motor test, tapping each finger to her thumb as fast as she could. The report also included an interview with Steve and Maggie Kaufman, with footage that Maggie had taken of Steve as he built the sprawling back deck. Finally, Bob, Elaine, and Kristen Suthers appeared live with Diane Sawyer in the studio.

Bob wore a tan sport coat, a white shirt and tie. Elaine sat to his left, her hands folded in her lap, wearing a lime green jacket and black slacks. Kristen sat to her left and wore a black dress suit. Ms. Sawyer first asked Bob about his condition prior to GDNF. Bob, visibly nervous, stammered that walking—walking had got to be such a problem. That changed on GDNF.

"I could walk into town," he said. "But now I'm so limited in what I can do because I can't walk even, and I know as this progresses it's only going to get worse."

Ms. Sawyer turned to Elaine and asked what she thought about Amgen's claim that Bob's improvements were the result of placebo effect.

"I've been a nurse for almost 50 years. I've seen placebo effect," she said. "I live with this man. This was not placebo effect. He had been on placebo for the first half of the study, all through last winter, and nothing happened. We knew he was not getting it. He became better as he got the GDNF gradually—it was very gradual, almost imperceptible . . . but we could see it so clearly, Diane."

Ms. Sawyer looked at Kristen and asked about the health risks of continuing GDNF. Kristen replied that GDNF had not caused any damage in the monkeys until it was abruptly taken away.

Ms. Sawyer then turned to Bob: "So, what you want most, Mr. Suthers, is to be able to make your choice, even if you know you're making a choice toward risk? You want to make the choice?"

"Oh yes, I want the GDNF. Definitely that's what I want. I want the GDNF—if I could say that into the camera [he looks at the camera]. That's what I want, the GDNF."

Ms. Sawyer asked Elaine why Amgen would shelve such a promising treatment. Elaine answered that she suspected the company had become skittish during the controversies surrounding pain drugs Vioxx and Celebrex.

"But you know you can't throw the baby out with the bathwater," Elaine continued. "They have a very wonderful drug that will help thousands and thousands of Parkinson's patients, and they just need to take ethical responsibility, both to this group of patients and to those they haven't treated yet. And we know they will. They couldn't possibly not, after we've sent so many testimonials."

27 Victory

As the meeting between the FDA and the investigators neared, Amgen had good reason to believe that the FDA would frown on any attempts to restart the GDNF trials. On August 26, 2004, when the company had just gotten word about the brain damaged monkeys and was deliberating whether to pull the plug, Amgen had contacted the FDA to explain its reasons for doing so. In a letter sent out to investigators on the day the trials ended, Amgen's Donna Masterman stated that the company had received the support of the FDA and the equivalent agencies in England and Canada. "This decision has been reviewed with the FDA, Health Canada and the Medicines and Healthcare Products regulatory Agency in the U.K. and they have all agreed with our recommendations," Dr. Masterman stated in the letter.

Four months later, the investigators who fought for the trials to resume hoped they could persuade the FDA not to interfere. There were really two questions to answer: Could those who once received GDNF have it back, and could Amgen resume its development of GDNF with new trials that would involve new patients?

The meeting took place on January 11, 2005. The investigators knew their 3 P.M. meeting with the FDA might be their patients' only shot at recovering GDNF. They met at 10 A.M. in the Ramada Inn, just a few blocks from the FDA administration building in Rockville, Maryland; and they practiced their presentation. It was a bit rough the first time through, but they polished it and came to a final agreement about the order of the PowerPoint slides.

They ate lunch at an Italian restaurant nearby with some employees from Medtronic. Medtronic was interested in acquiring the rights to GDNF, or at least the rights to deliver it by pump. The company had an interest in making the delivery method work since it was, after all, a Medtronic pump that squirted GDNF through a Medtronic catheter into the patients' brains. If the pump-and-catheter method could be refined and proved effective, the company would have a de facto monopoly on the required hardware when the therapy went to market. The company's goals aligned well with the Kentucky doctors' desires to resume the trials. After lunch, the group entered the concrete and glass administration building for the 3 P.M. meeting.

According to the FDA's official minutes of the meeting, it included seven FDA officials, eight Amgen employees, three Medtronic employees, and five investigators, including Dr. Penn from Chicago and Drs. Gash and Gerhardt from Kentucky. The investigators who supported Amgen decision—the doctors from Toronto, Oregon, Virginia, and Duke University—were absent. The minutes state that the Amgen contingent said it would take a back seat in the discussion: "Amgen's stated role in the meeting was to listen to the investigators and the agency, to provide support for the discussion (with factual information), and facilitate the meeting, as required."

At this point, Dr. Gash later said in an interview, Chicago's Dr. Penn interjected and asked if Amgen would also be willing to take a literal back seat and move toward the back of the room so the five investigators could sit up front, face to face with the seven FDA officials. According to Dr. Gash, the Amgen and Medtronic employees rose and obliged. Dr. Penn's request set the tone for the meeting: this was a discussion between the FDA and the investigators.

The investigator's presentation focused on the two chief safety concerns: the brain damage in the monkeys and the antibodies that had turned up in five patients. The investigators had invited John S. Thompson, an immunologist from the University of Kentucky, to discuss the antibody issue. According to Dr. Gash, Thompson said the antibodies were a concern and should be monitored closely but that so far there had been no adverse symptoms reported in the patients who had them.

The time then turned to Dr. Gash, who discussed the brain damage in the monkeys. He later recalled, "I pointed out [the dose of GDNF in the damaged monkeys] was a very, very high dose. We had not seen it in any other animals or any patients. . . . We hadn't seen any evidence of that from high-resolution MRI scans. The pathology indicated the brain damage was a one-time event, that it was not progressive."

Dr. Gash told the FDA he believed that the unusually high dose of GDNF, followed by its abrupt withdrawal, had caused the brain damage. He knew that of the four monkeys, only three had been withdrawn *intentionally* after six months. But he believed it was very possible that the fourth monkey's pump had malfunctioned at some point during the six-month study, which would have created a similar, though unintentional, abrupt withdrawal. "I said, 'From my experience with the pumps, you can have a number of reasons why delivery stops,'" Dr. Gash recalled.

After the investigators had presented, they asked for the FDA's perspective on the trials. FDA officials described their first conversations with Amgen, in late August of 2004, when the Amgen had proposed halting the GDNF trials. The official minutes summarize the FDA's position at the time this way: "The agency's approach was that if the data did not clearly direct what 'the correct' action would be, then it was the company's prerogative how to proceed. Amgen's choice [to halt the trials] was one of a number of reasonable possibilities."

This assessment must have pleased the Amgen representatives in the room. The FDA had stated that the company's decision to stop the trials was reasonable. The next paragraph of the minutes, however, shows that the FDA was not convinced GDNF had caused the brain damage directly. "The agency agrees with the investigators that there is not presently a good understanding of the mechanism that is the basis of the monkey toxicity." Hearing this must have been encouraging to the investigators in the room: the FDA was actually acknowledging the possibility of abrupt withdrawal as the cause of the brain damage.

The FDA officials said that because the safety issues were unresolved, it would not be appropriate to give GDNF to new patients. But the FDA also made clear that it would not interfere if Amgen decided to give the drug back to the patients who already had received it: "As far as the withdrawal of the product from clinical trials is concerned, the agency has not controlled what has happened. The decision to withdraw was, and remains, a decision made by Amgen. . . .

"In some prior situations with other drugs, when a drug has been discontinued, a company may have chosen to allow patients that are already receiving drug to continue to do so for an extended period of time, and . . . the FDA has often permitted such proposals to go forth. . . . After patient re-consent, continued administration has been allowed in those patients who personally feel they have benefited from the drug and have shown an absence of marked apparent drug-related adverse effects.

"If continued studies are to be pursued with the experienced patients, it is important to ensure there is well-coordinated, ongoing safety monitoring of the patients, and that all parties do what is feasible to monitor for the existing safety uncertainties."

And just like that, the FDA had given the green light to resume GDNF testing under carefully monitored conditions. According to several of the investigators present, Amgen's representatives at the meeting appeared surprised at the FDA's position. Amgen's Dr. Masterman had been certain that the FDA would forbid the company from giving GDNF back to the patients. Now, the agency had cleared the way for just that.

"They were shocked," Dr. Gash said. "You could read it on their faces."

The day after the meeting, Dr. Gerhardt from Kentucky participated in a telephone conference call with officials from the Parkinson's Action Network. He reported on what was discussed in the meeting and on the FDA's position that Amgen could resume the trials if it so chose. To those who had been fighting to return GDNF to the patients, it was excellent news.

Perry Cohen had been following the development of GDNF for years. The non-profit group he heads, the Parkinson Pipeline Project, is a grassroots organization that monitors emerging therapies and pushes for more patient involvement in the way companies develop drugs and how the government regulates them. Mr. Cohen was diagnosed with Parkinson's in 1996 and has been deeply involved in Parkinson's treatment development and advocacy ever since. The Pipeline Project supported the patients early on in the GDNF controversy and remained involved during the following years. (For example, it was at the Pipeline Project's booth in Washington D.C. where I first saw the before-and-after videos of the Bristol patients.)

Mr. Cohen was on the conference call when Dr. Gerhardt described the FDA meeting, and he sent an e-mail to Maggie Kaufman, Kristen Suthers, and a handful of others to share the good news.

"It is still up to Amgen whether to provide the treatment for extended use," Mr. Cohen wrote. "In my discussions with Amgen they have taken a position that patient safety is the sole primary reason for halting the development of this method to deliver GDNF, and when asked they indicated no financial calculations entered into the decision. So the result of yesterday's hearing would mean that Amgen has no barrier to supply the medicine as they had promised when they recruited the 50 patients into this risky study. As advocates we should now give Amgen the opportunity to make good on its promises."

It was far from a victory cry. Mr. Cohen was simply following the facts to their logical conclusion: If patient safety had been Amgen's only obstacle to resuming the trials, and if that obstacle now had been removed, it would follow that Amgen would have no reason to withhold GDNF any longer. As the recipients of Mr. Cohen's e-mail forwarded it on to friends and colleagues, it spurred many excited questions. Was Amgen going to return GDNF? Or was it just that the company now had sole discretion to do so? Either way, it was an excellent sign for the patients in any case. The FDA was not going to interfere.

Mr. Cohen didn't know the answer to those questions. He was as anxious as anyone to know what Amgen's next move would be. Mr. Cohen later said it was at this point that he answered an unexpected phone call from an Amgen's co-leader of the GDNF project: "Mike Reilly called me out of the blue and started telling me how Amgen was going to give GDNF for compassionate use, but they needed a couple of weeks to determine who could have their pumps restarted because it might be dangerous to restart pumps if they hadn't been running with the saline solution. . . . I couldn't sit on that news so I sent e-mails to people I know giving the facts as I understood them."

Mr. Cohen sent out another e-mail the next day, and this time he left little room for doubt: the patients had scored a major victory.

> I received a call from [Amgen's] Mike Reilly who confirmed our understanding of the FDA opinion shown in the prior email . . . Amgen will spend a week or two to establish criteria to determine eligibility for the extended use. The company will then work with study doctors to establish a new protocol, including procedures for counseling patients, and each patient in consultation with his doctor will assess the risks and benefits of continuing on the medicine. In other words we get what we wanted for the study participants!!!! He asked us to be patient while they implement this, and I asked that patients be asked to participate in determining criteria for continued access. Good news!!

The news came as a shock to Kristen Suthers. Despite the confidence that her mother had expressed to Diane Sawyer on *Good Morning America* that Amgen would reconsider, she had serious doubts that Amgen would ever return the drug. She had made so many phone calls and sent so many letters with no indication of a change in the status quo. And yet, Perry Cohen's message was clear. Amgen planned to give GDNF back to her father. She, her family, and her friends had fought the world's largest biotechnology company—and won!

She sent her own summary of the good news to her contacts in the United States and England: "Amgen called Perry Cohen and told him they were willing to provide GDNF on a compassionate basis to all the study participants! . . . There are still logistics to work out, but it looks really good. In reality I will believe it when I see Dad on the exam table getting the injections—but at this point, all signs say it will happen. I am in shock!"

The good news ricocheted around the internet on blogs and message boards. A rag-tag group of patients and their doctors had challenged the world's biggest biotech company and prevailed—a fairytale ending. Donna Masterman, co-leader of the GDNF project at Amgen, got wind of the Web rumors and alerted her colleague Michael Reilly. The two called Perry Cohen and told him that he must have misunderstood Mr. Reilly's earlier statements over the phone. Mr. Reilly later recalled of that second conversation: "I said, 'Perry, that's not what I said to you.' I said, 'We're *considering* this issue, and we haven't made a decision on it yet.'

Perry Cohen maintains that Mr. Reilly was quite clear in the first phone call.

Mr. Cohen communicated this conversation to the other patients, doctors and advocates. It was demoralizing and potentially embarrassing news. Some had sounded the victory cry to extended family and friends. Kristen Suthers had sent an e-mail to dozens of supporters who had helped in a letter-writing campaign. She, Maggie Kaufman and Tom Isaacs let their friends and family know it had been a false alarm.

28 Final Decision

The already high profile of the GDNF issue in the patient and research communities continued to grow after Amgen's meeting with the FDA and the investigators. On January 28, 2005 the Parkinson's Action Network issued a statement urging Amgen to return GDNF to the patients and to continue to develop the drug. On February 6, the New York City-based Parkinson's Disease Foundation released a similar statement.

Weeks passed without any formal response from the company. Amgen's Michael Reilly later described Amgen's internal deliberations this way:

> The whole [GDNF] team was involved and, yes, there were discussions in rooms of 20 people, maybe, and yes, both the head of R&D [Roger Perlmutter] . . . and the CEO of the company [Kevin Sharer] personally asked each person, personally sought opposing points of view—and there *were* opposing points of view. And there were people who flipped their minds back and forth between the two views during

> the four months. It was that process internally and reaching out externally to decide whether in fact we were going to stay with that decision or change it.

Before joining Amgen, Roger Perlmutter was overseeing basic research at Merck, and after joining Amgen in January of 2001 he recruited a number of his top-level colleagues at Merck to come work for him at Amgen. Perlmutter had overseen the development of Vioxx, and when Merck ordered the drug pulled from the market in late September of 2004, it is reasonable to assume that Perlmutter and the other former Merck employees at Amgen took notice. (Merck was accused of painting too rosy a picture of its blockbusting painkiller Vioxx, which independent studies showed increased likelihood of a heart attack.) Vioxx users sued Merck by the thousands. The company's stock plunged 40 percent. The Vioxx scandal ballooned throughout the fall and into the winter, and it coincided with Amgen's internal deliberations over whether to return GDNF to the patients.

Mr. Reilly said talk of the mounting Vioxx scandal entered into the discussions only superficially. The GDNF team members sometimes would muse at the irony that drug companies apparently could do nothing right. On the one hand there was GDNF, a drug patients said was too valuable to be shelved. On the other was Vioxx, a drug suddenly criticized for being too harmful to sell. "It was this 'damned if you do, damned if you don't' type of thing," Mr. Reilly said.

The FDA had cleared the way for Amgen to give GDNF back to the patients, but a month went by and Amgen still had not given an answer. The answer finally came on Friday, February 12, 2005. The answer was no.

It is a common public relation strategy to release controversial or unpopular information late in the day on a Friday. Television stations don't have enough time to put a story together for Friday's evening news, and newspapers print the story in the less-read Saturday paper. Amgen sent press releases to major media outlets and to a few patient organizations. The GDNF patients got the news as it filtered down to them by e-mail and telephone. Amgen had decided to deny compassionate use of GDNF.

Don Gash said he and the other investigators from Kentucky learned of Amgen's decision through patient groups that had seen Amgen's press release. Later in the day, Dr. Gash joined a conference call with six Amgen employees and the lead investigators from Bristol, Chicago and NYU. A transcript of the conversation reveals how vigorous the debate over GDNF reinstatement had become.

On the line, Roger Perlmutter began gingerly. "Over the last several months we have agonized over this," he said. "I've had the opportunity to speak with many of you personally. We've also reached out to investigators skilled in clinical trials in Parkinson's disease, to bioethicists, and we've examined all the data internally and tried to come to the right decision. I can't tell you how agonizing this has been for all of us."

Then he said the words the investigators knew were coming: "At the end of the day we have decided not to re-administer GDNF to 48 patients who have previously been exposed to it out of concern for patient well being."

He followed the words with a lengthy description of the myriad factors the company had considered—the apparent success of the early trials, the failure of the most recent one, the antibodies, the monkeys, and so on. He expressed sympathy to the investigators, who he knew were dealing with the patients directly. "We are devastated that GDNF did not work in this trial. We wish so much that we could offer them an effective therapy, but instead, we just offer them our support and our hope for the future," he said. "With that,

I'm happy to take questions that you might have. Of course, I know there's a lot of concern out there."

Dr. Penn from Chicago, who had been instrumental in arranging the meeting with the FDA, interjected: "I might lead since I was the one that went to the FDA and got their permission for you people to start up again. As the FDA says, they certainly don't control the drug, but you people do. Would you consider allowing the patent rights for that type of delivery of GDNF to be given to a third party, if they are willing to investigate it? If not, why not? Because that means you're just using your monopoly to make sure, on your judgment, that we don't use the drug on these patients."

Dr. Penn's pointed questions must have been rather jarring against Dr. Perlmutter's elegant introduction. Dr. Perlmutter began to respond circuitously. "Well, I think that's a dialogue that we should have . . ." he began, and spoke of various issues that had come up during the phase II trial. "Initially when we got these results there was certainly the feeling from Steve Gill and Don Gash in part that the catheter administration was incorrect and that this catheter wouldn't work because everything was tracking back."

"Do you mind me interrupting?" Dr. Penn cut in. "I'm asking a very simple question. Why won't you allow a third party to use the GDNF the way that might be appropriate for the patients?"

Dr. Penn didn't get his answer until several minutes later, after the conversation had grown more contentious. The other investigators on the line, Drs. Gash, Gill, and Hutchinson, had questioned Dr. Perlmutter about flaws in the design of the phase II trial and about the possibility of withdrawal phenomenon. Finally, Dr. Penn cut in with, "Instead of arguing about all of this we have to find out whether Amgen is willing to consider another pathway out of this difficulty."

"We are not," Dr. Perlmutter replied.

"You are not. This has to do with your morally knowing that it's better not to do this because you've made that judgment," Dr. Penn challenged.

"Based on discussions with an enormous number of people, I'm sure of our data," Dr. Perlmutter countered.

"So that is—period—how you stand? So there's no sense in discussing this with you any more since it's an immutable position."

"It's an immutable position."

"Well, it is. I mean, in the sense that our patients are not going to receive this drug from Amgen in time to treat their disease in a reasonable way."

"I would point out that I don't believe that GDNF can treat their disease."

"I understand that, but that's your opinion and not the patients' and some doctors' opinions. But others agree with you wholeheartedly. That's fine, but it does suggest to me that you're making a judgment that you think is right for everybody. And there is no way of getting away from the fact that you own [GDNF] and you [won't] allow anybody else to do it. I mean, you have the poison sitting there, from your standpoint, and you don't want anybody else to have the poison. And since you control it, you're not going to let anybody have the poison. Other people feel that it isn't poison. So we're not going to get anywhere unless you allow other people to investigate it."

Dr. Perlmutter stood his ground, and deflected challenges from Drs. Hutchinson and Gash about the toxicology data. After several minutes, he said, "Of course, the easy thing to do is say, 'Sure, what the hell, let's give it to them.' We're taking a much harder road here."

Dr. Penn responded: "You're taking what is the moral road from your standpoint, where you've decided that the facts are the way they are. But there is discussion as to what really is the case, and the FDA is allowing that. So I don't see any impediment to your recognizing that you might not be right. Okay, and it's a pretty hard thing to do as a company."

"Reasonable people can disagree and do disagree about many aspects of this. We've chosen under the circumstances to fall on the side of safety," Dr. Perlmutter said.

"That's fine. You've chosen that and made it impossible for anybody else to do further investigation other than Amgen in the way that you want to do it. So you're sitting basically on a monopoly on this investigation."

The call ended shortly thereafter.

29 The Lawyer

Kristen Suthers didn't wait long to look for an attorney. When she learned Amgen had denied compassionate use of GDNF, she concluded that the only way to recover the drug for her father would be through the courts. She searched online for the names of attorneys who had represented patients in clinical trial disputes. One name surfaced again and again: Alan C. Milstein.

Mr. Milstein was an attorney at the New Jersey firm Sherman, Silverstein, Kohl, Rose and Podolsky, and he had argued several high-profile cases in recent years. One profile of Mr. Milstein, published in the December 30, 2001 edition of the *Washington Post Magazine*, seemed especially encouraging. The illustration on the magazine's cover shows an armor-clad knight on a horse, lance drawn, riding at a full gallop across an empty, serene plain toward a city far in the distance. In bold, black letters below the knight is the cover story's title, "The Crusader."

The profile, written by New York-based journalist Jennifer Washburn, chronicles Mr. Milstein's circuitous route to law and his eventual ascent to become "the man to see when it comes to medical research abuses." He grew up in a middle-class Baltimore suburb. His father ran a liquor store and his mother was a homemaker. He embraced the counterculture of the 1950s and 1960s (and still keeps a picture of Bob Dylan on his office wall). After graduating from the University of Maryland in 1975, he earned a master's degree in American studies at the University of Kansas and then worked as an art critic for a small newspaper in Philadelphia. After the birth of his first child, Mr. Milstein realized his newspaper job wasn't going to pay the bills. He attended law school at Temple University in Philadelphia and later joined Sherman, Silverstein, Kohl, Rose and Podolsky in 1991. He spent the following years specializing in insurance, computer software, and product liability litigation.

Then in December 1999, a longtime client of the firm brought his brother, Paul Gelsinger, a contractor from Tucson, to discuss the death of Paul's son, Jesse. Jesse had died three months earlier during a gene therapy experiment at the University of Pennsylvania that was designed to help find a cure for a genetic liver disorder.

Jesse's own condition was already effectively controlled through medication and a special diet, but he had been led to believe that Penn's investigators were close to finding a cure for infants who suffered a more deadly form of Jesse's disease. He believed that his participation would move the science forward, so he entered the trial. According to the *Washington Post Magazine,* the experiment went terribly wrong: "The large dose of genetically engineered viruses that researchers infused into Jesse's liver in September 1999 caused a massive reaction. His liver failed, his blood thickened into jelly, and his kidneys, brain and other vital organs shut down. Four days after the initial infusion he was brain-dead. His death was the first reported fatality in the gene therapy field—a much-vaunted new science with heavy Wall Street financing—and made international headlines."

Though Paul Gelsinger initially defended the scientists at Penn, he eventually began to doubt that the investigators had been forthright about the risks of the trial. That's when he approached Mr. Milstein. At that point, Mr. Milstein had never argued a medical malpractice case, and he had no experience litigating against research institutions. What began as a favor to a longtime client, however, evolved into a personal crusade. Mr. Milstein studied the long and disturbing history of human experimentation. He saw a connection between Jesse Gelsinger's case and the infamous experiments of the past, such as those conducted on Jews, Gypsies, and the mentally ill during the Holocaust and the infamous Tuskegee experiment conducted between 1932 and 1972 in the United States, in which a potentially saving treatment was intentionally withheld from black men so that government researchers could observe the effects of the disease.

The University of Pennsylvania settled the Gelsinger case for an undisclosed amount that is believed to be between $5 million and $10 million. The case also brought sweeping ethics reforms to the university after it was discovered that some of the investigators involved in the botched gene therapy trial stood to profit financially if it succeeded.

To Kristen Suthers, Mr. Milstein was the obvious choice. She needed someone who would not be intimidated by the immense resources and the army of attorneys that Amgen would have at its disposal. Mr. Milstein had represented patients and their families in cases that pitted him against major research institutions, and he had won. She contacted his office and started to tell the GDNF story. He and the firm agreed to take on the case. It would cost the patients nothing unless they won.

30 The Lawsuit

When Alan Milstein filed a lawsuit against Amgen Inc. on behalf of Bob Suthers and another NYU patient named Niwana Martin, he was venturing into new and rather unusual territory, at least for him. By that time, he had several years of experience representing clinical trial participants. Where his previous clients sought restitution for having been harmed during a clinical trial, however, his new clients were claiming just the opposite—that GDNF had helped them and that Amgen had harmed patients by taking it away.

The lawsuit claimed that Amgen had agreed both verbally and in writing to provide GDNF indefinitely, so long as the drug was safe and effective. By halting the trials and withholding GDNF, the suit alleged, the company had violated the terms of these agreements. Attached to the lawsuits were sworn statements from six former GDNF patients and the lead investigators from New York, Chicago, and Kentucky. The patients universally testified to the effectiveness of GDNF. In his affidavit, Bob Suthers stated that he had "expected to continue receiving doses of the drug indefinitely" and that he "experienced significant improvement after receiving GDNF." Niwana Martin and the other patients testified similarly.

"I had significantly more 'on' time, felt physically, cognitively and emotionally better, was able to take less other medication, lost my facial mask, enjoyed an improved sense of smell and began to be able to walk, and sometimes even run, without restrictions or impediments, once I was on GDNF," Ms. Martin stated.[41]

The investigators' statements were universally critical of Amgen's decision to stop the trials. "I, along with other principal investigators, believed, and still believe, that GDNF was safe and of benefit to the plaintiffs," Dr. Hutchinson stated. "Since GDNF was withdrawn, Mr. Suthers has been confused easily, has had serious language difficulties, has had serious walking difficulty, can no longer bathe himself, has suffered from increased tremors, and can only walk one-quarter of a mile per day, as opposed to two miles per day while he was on GDNF. Similarly, all of the improvements that Ms. Martin showed during the period that she was on GDNF are gone. The decision by Amgen to terminate the trial was unreasonable and contrary to its fiduciary and contractual obligations to the plaintiffs." Dr. Penn from Chicago and the research team from Kentucky gave similar statements.

On the same day he filed the lawsuit, Mr. Milstein filed a "preliminary injunction" that demanded immediate access to GDNF until the lawsuit was resolved. The case might drag on for months or years, but the injunction would ensure that Bob Suthers and Niwana Martin received GDNF in the meantime. In order for the preliminary injunction to be successful, Mr. Milstein would first have to demonstrate to a judge that the lawsuit itself has a reasonable likelihood of success. He would also need to show that his clients would likely suffer irreparable injury without the injunction.

The judge's decision regarding the preliminary injunction would be very telling about the patient's overall chance of success in the lawsuit. The judge would need to decide whether or not Amgen had a legal obligation to provide GDNF, assuming that the drug was safe and effective. Then he would need to decide, based on the evidence, whether GDNF *was* safe and effective and whether the patients were likely to suffer irreparable injury without it. If he rejected either of these claims from the start, it would not bode well for the patients' case.

About three weeks after Mr. Milstein filed the lawsuit and the injunction, Amgen responded by filing a 33-page brief that urged the court to deny the injunction. The company argued that, contrary to the plaintiff's claims, Amgen had absolutely no obligation to provide GDNF to the patients: "Far from promising an indefinite supply of GDNF, the clear language of the informed consent document expressly provides that Amgen has the right to do exactly what it has done—i.e., terminate the study. . . ."

Filed along with this brief were 26 documents in support, including statements from several Amgen employees and from the lead investigators from Oregon, Toronto, North Carolina, and Virginia.

Up to this point, Amgen had said relatively little publicly about its internal deliberation on halting the trial or allowing compassionate use. The new statements provided some insight into how the company arrived at its conclusion and why Amgen was unwilling to make an exception for the 48 patients who had received GDNF. In a 13-page sworn affidavit, Amgen's Roger Perlmutter, described the reasons for ending the trials in September of 2004: "Amgen employed a risk-benefit analysis in determining whether to halt the phase II studies. The benefit factor was zero, because the unblinding of the study revealed no efficacy of GDNF as compared to placebo. Any risk, weighed against a lack of any benefit at all, would weigh in favor of not continuing the study. In this case the risks were grave. . . .

"I participated in making that decision. It was a decision that, while painful, was absolutely clear based upon the clinical evidence. All GDNF team members agreed with the decision."

He also described the company's reasons for denying compassionate use in February of 2005: "Continuing to provide GDNF could create false hope and deter patients from pursuing potentially helpful therapies that are already approved by the FDA. . . . If Amgen were to supply GDNF to the patients, the placebo effect would likely persist, and false hope would be created for a community that would also want GDNF."

He went on to say that by making an exception and granting compassionate use for the 48 GDNF patients Amgen would undermine the scientific process by which it produces saving therapies. "Amgen needs to be consistent in its approach to developing therapies that treat grievous illness. This will not be the last time that Amgen endeavors to develop a therapy for patients with devastating illness, and this will probably not be the last time Amgen fails to achieve it. As a company, Amgen cannot hold each drug and disease to a different standard.

"Amgen is a responsible company that has a rigorous scientific process in place for a reason. If the company deviated from that process in any one case, the integrity of the process is compromised."

Other Amgen employees weighed in similarly. Donna Masterman, who co-led the GDNF team, wrote that "Amgen feels strongly that 'putting patients first' means it cannot ethically continue to expose patients to [pump-delivered] GDNF, given the serious safety concerns and absence of any proven benefit."

The lawsuit made clear the division between the investigators at the eight trial sites. Roughly half of them cooperated with Mr.

Milstein and provided statements in support of the lawsuits, and the other half cooperated with Amgen's lawyers and provided statements in support of the company. Only Dr. Gill, the lead investigator from Bristol, remained aloof. He provided no statement to either side.

In a statement on behalf of Amgen, Dr. Frederick Wooten from the University of Virginia stated, "I believe Amgen's decision to terminate the open-label study and to discontinue GDNF dosing of study subjects was appropriate, well-justified, and made in good faith based upon scientific evidence. I very much support Amgen's decision to discontinue the study."

The four pro-Amgen investigators also challenged the notion that Amgen had committed to provide GDNF indefinitely. Tony Lang, the lead investigator for the site in Toronto, stated, "At no time did I understand, nor did I or my colleagues convey to study subjects enrolled at Toronto Western Hospital, that Amgen would continue to provide GDNF to study participants indefinitely, regardless of the safety and efficacy data received and evaluated by Amgen. It was my understanding that Amgen retained the right to terminate the study."

The case was assigned to District Judge H. Kevin Castel and a preliminary hearing was scheduled for May 26, 2005. The hearing would give attorneys from both sides a forum to present their arguments. Both sides agreed that rather than call witnesses to testify at the hearing, they would rely on the many written testimonies that already had been filed with the court. Whatever Judge Castel decided regarding the request for the preliminary injunction, the ruling would be a good indicator of how the lawsuit would fare at trial—or if it would even get that far.

31 GDNF in Court

On May 26, 2005, the Suthers family and Mr. Milstein arrived at the Daniel Patrick Moynihan U.S. Courthouse at 500 Pearl Street in downtown New York City. The soaring concrete structure was dedicated and named for the former New York senator in 2000 by then Mayor Rudy Giuliani, and it had since housed the operations of the federal district court for the Southern District of New York.

The hearing began promptly at 10 A.M. Mr. Milstein sat with his co-counsel, an attorney named Michael Dube who worked with him at the firm. Across the aisle sat one woman and two men who would represent Amgen. The company had hired Hogan and Hartson LLP, the largest Washington D.C.-based firm, to represent them in the GDNF matter. A man named Mark D. Gately was Amgen's lead counsel. He shared a common heritage with his colleague across the aisle: both he and Mr. Milstein were born and raised in Baltimore and both received their undergraduate degrees at the University of Maryland. Mr. Gately continued at the university for his law degree and, after graduating in 1977, began to distinguish himself as a competent trial lawyer.

The audience rose and Judge Castel entered. After exchanging quick pleasantries with attorneys from both sides, he gave the time to Mr. Milstein to present his argument. The hearing would allow each side to argue for or against the preliminary injunction. Mr. Milstein, rising from his seat, began.

"Your honor, this case is of profound importance—on the macro level because it affects the rights of research subjects in future medical research, and on the micro level because it affects the lives of two individuals who are profoundly ill and who need GDNF in order to live."[42]

Mr. Milstein would need to clear two legal hurdles to win GDNF for his clients. First, he would need to show that their lawsuit had a good chance of succeeding, which meant proving that Amgen promised to provide the drug indefinitely if it were safe and effective. Second, he would have to show that his clients needed the drug urgently, that they would suffer irreparable harm without it. If he failed to prove the first point, the judge wouldn't even consider the second. And if he proved the first but not the second, his clients wouldn't get the drug back.

He continued: "Now, the real question here is, does the drug work? Everything that Amgen said in its papers is predicated on the conclusion that it doesn't work, because if it doesn't work, no risk is worth 'no benefit.' Without benefit, any risk tips in favor of stopping the trial.

"Without benefit, there's no promise or duty to provide it," he said. "There is no irreparable harm if you don't get it."

Judge Castel interrupted before Mr. Milstein went much further. Before he looked at whether or not GDNF works, the judge said, he wanted to know what documents or promises obligated Amgen to provide GDNF. "I have to find the existence of a contract," he said. "I have to find probability of success on the merits before I even consider the question of irreparable harm."

Mr. Milstein pointed to the statements given by Dr. Hutchinson and by his clients, the patients. The patients had testified that they expected to receive GDNF indefinitely, provided it was safe and effective. Dr. Hutchinson stated that his patients had every right to expect this and that Amgen had confirmed as much to him in a telephone conversation. Mr. Milstein also directed the judge to the 22-page informed consent document that all the NYU patients signed before enrolling in the original six-month trial. One passage told patients that "the principal investigator may also decide to withdraw you from the study under certain circumstances. Some possible reasons for withdrawing the subject from the study would be deteriorating health or other conditions that might make continued participation harmful to you."

"What does the informed consent document say?" Mr. Milstein continued. "That promise says the principal investigator—it's going to be his decision as to whether or not to terminate their participation in the trial."

Judge Castel asked Mr. Milstein to explain how a commitment from NYU or from Dr. Hutchinson amounted to a commitment from Amgen. In response, Mr. Milstein described the relationship between the drug company that sponsors a trial and the researchers who carry it out.

"Amgen can't conduct the clinical trials inside its building with its doctors because it has a conflict of interest. It has an interest in getting its drug to market, having its stock price go up, having its revenues increased. And so it needs to step back and let independent principal investigators conduct the research, to let their safety monitoring boards evaluate the data from the research, have

[Institutional Review Boards] review whether the research is ethical and whether it's being conducted ethically," he said. "Everybody outside of Amgen, at least with respect to these plaintiffs, believed that the drug was safe and effective and the trial should go on."

It was inappropriate, Mr. Milstein argued, for Amgen to give control of the trial to NYU initially and then to halt the trial without consulting with the university or with the lead investigator. Dr. Hutchinson and NYU had made promises to the patients based on Amgen's instructions, Mr. Milstein said, and so a commitment from NYU or Dr. Hutchinson was in essence a commitment from Amgen.

Judge Castel said, "Well, let me ask you, is Hutchinson Amgen, in your view?"

"Is Hutchinson Amgen?"

"In your view," said the judge.

"Yes."

"All right. How do you square that with what you just described for me a minute ago about the importance to Amgen of having an independent researcher with no affiliation because they can't do this research on their own because they're conflicted; they need independent entities to conduct the research?"

Mr. Milstein said, "They do. And he was an independent entity to conduct the research. But in the patients' eyes—they don't see Amgen. Amgen has set up this research enterprise, and they have set it up in a way that they have placed Dr. Hutchinson as their only representative in the enterprise. He's the one who provides them with the informed consent document. He's the one who has read the protocol and discusses it with them. He's the one who gives them the drug. He's the one who makes the promises. If they have questions, he talks to Amgen. . . . He says, 'Is this what we're going to do?' And then he communicates back to the patients.

"And he says, based on what I told these patients, they had reason to believe—and contracts are all about reasonable expectations—they had reason to believe that if the drug were safe and effective, Amgen would continue to supply it."

After a few more minutes of argument, Mr. Milstein sat down and the Judge Castel asked to hear from Mr. Gately. He had authorized Mr. Milstein and Mr. Gately to appear in the court *pro hac vice,* a legal term that means an attorney can practice temporarily in a court to which he or she has not been formally admitted. As he began, Mr. Gately's ingratiating manner contrasted with Mr. Milstein's frank, aggressive approach.

"May it please the court, your honor, Mark Gately for the defendant Amgen," he began. "I want to thank you for allowing me to appear in the court *pro hac vice,* and I want to thank the court for the time you spent going through the voluminous materials which we've supplied to you."

Mr. Gately would need to convince the court of two things: first, that the lawsuit against Amgen had little chance of success, and second, that the patients weren't likely to suffer irreparable harm as a result. He began first by addressing the lawsuit—the patients' claims of breach of contract and so on.

Amgen's argument was simple: there was no contract. There was no scrap of paper that showed any type of agreement between the company and the patients. The only relevant agreement had been between Amgen and the research institution, and that agreement stated Amgen could halt the trial "immediately upon written notice."

That might have settled the question about a written contract, but the patients also had claimed *promissory estoppel,* a legal doctrine that holds that even non-written promises can be enforced. Under the right circumstances, even verbal promises can be legally binding.

The patients claimed that Amgen had promised—through Dr. Hutchinson—to continue to provide the drug indefinitely. To refute the claim, Mr. Gately would need to demonstrate that Amgen made no such promises.

"Amgen had no relationship with these individuals," Mr. Gately told the court. "There's no evidence that Amgen ever had any dealings with these people. . . . Clearly, Dr. Hutchinson is not an agent of Amgen. In fact, the documents themselves say that. They say that the investigators are not agents, that they're independent contractors. And New York law, as we cited in our brief, does not allow someone to invest themselves with apparent agency powers. So there is nothing to show any agreement between Amgen and these individuals in the study. Nothing in writing, nothing orally from Amgen."

Mr. Gately next turned his attention to the matter of irreparable harm: Would Bob Suthers and Niwana Martin suffer irreparable harm without GDNF?

"On the irreparable harm side, your honor, there are numerous cases which we've cited which say, where a drug does not have proven efficacy, there can't be irreparable harm. We are also here nine to ten months, if I'm counting right, after this drug was stopped. And you're being asked to find that there was immediate irreparable harm, which is somewhat of a strange situation after the passage of time. Why is it irreparable harm now?"

In other words, whatever harm the withdrawal of GDNF might cause should already be evident in these patients. And while both Bob Suthers and Niwana Martin had stated that their symptoms were slowly returning, it would be hard to prove that in court.

"After all the discussion and after all of the passion and heartache that's connected with this case on all sides, we really come down to the basic first-year law school issues. There wasn't a contract here. The likelihood of success on the merits is not overwhelmingly strong. It's not strong at all. It's very weak to nonexistent. Their irreparable harm argument, when one looks at all of the factors, particularly the safety signals, does not meet the standard for mandatory injunction. And the injunction should be denied here, your honor."

He thanked Judge Castel and sat, and then Mr. Milstein stood again for a brief rebuttal. By this time it had become clear that Amgen had the written evidence on its side. If Mr. Milstein's clients were to prevail, the court would need to understand that, regardless of what Amgen stated in writing, the company had led the patients to believe that if GDNF was safe and effective, they would get the drug indefinitely. From Mr. Milstein's point of view, the success of the patients' lawsuit hinged on whether GDNF worked. If it didn't work, there was no binding agreement and no reason to press on despite the safety concerns. Mr. Gately had argued simply that GDNF didn't work because in the phase II trial it performed no better than a placebo.

"Listen again to what [Mr. Gately] said time and time again," Mr. Milstein told the judge. "His argument really is, the stuff doesn't work. That's the way every one of those arguments work, because if the stuff doesn't work, there's no promise, there's no duty, there's no harm that would allow the court to issue this injunction."

He said in closing, "The promise was, if it works, and if I [speaking for Amgen] believe, by the principal investigator, that it's not risky to you, you'll get it. That's the implied, common-sense essence of this argument." He took his seat across the aisle from Mr. Gately, and Judge Castel said a few words in closing.

"All right. The matter is submitted. I think at the starting point it is clear to me, and both sides in their arguments have recognized this, that this case is really at bottom about two human beings, one,

Robert Suthers, and another, Niwana Martin. And certainly under the plaintiff's view of this case, the decision in this matter has real-life consequences to two human beings. And that alone makes it important."

The judge said he would promptly review the case. "I will endeavor to rule as quickly as I can, and I will issue a written decision."

32 Try, Try Again

The judge's decision came two weeks later, on June 6, 2005. His answer was to deny the preliminary injunction. He praised the patients for their courage in volunteering for such a demanding study, but he could find no evidence of any promise or contract between Amgen and the patients.

> [The] plaintiffs participated in research trials in GDNF in the utmost of good faith and with every hope for their success. It was in Amgen's financial interest that the research trials prove successful. In undertaking the trials, Amgen retained independent researchers to ensure that they were free from the influence of its own self-interest in the success of the trials. The independent researcher in this case, Dr. Hutchinson, presented to plaintiffs consent documents that acknowledged Amgen's right to terminate the research trials. Plaintiffs signed these documents and do not presently claim that they were coerced or misled into doing so. . . . The plaintiffs' motion for a preliminary injunction is denied.

The ruling was an enormous setback to the patients' case. Not only would they have to continue to wait for GDNF, but the judge's negative ruling also meant that he didn't think the suit was likely to succeed. Mr. Milstein and the patients decided to fight on anyway. Within three weeks of Judge Castel's denial, Mr. Milstein filed a lawsuit at the federal courthouse in downtown Lexington, Kentucky. This time the plaintiffs were eight of the nine Kentucky patients who had been receiving GDNF when the trials were halted. The parallel lawsuits would advance simultaneously. If one failed, the other might succeed.

The patients had reason to hope things would play out differently in Kentucky. The Kentucky patients had been part of a phase I trial that began in early 2002. That trial, unlike the later phase II trial, had produced dramatic results. It would be more difficult for Amgen to argue that GDNF hadn't benefited the Kentucky patients. Another crucial difference was in the wording of the key documents for the Kentucky trial. The informed consent agreement in New York had more or less made clear that Amgen could halt the trials at any time. The wording of the Kentucky documents was more vague, and one could argue that the Kentucky patients never knew Amgen had such authority.

As he had done before, Mr. Milstein filed a motion for a preliminary injunction along with the lawsuit, and as before, a hearing was scheduled to give each side an opportunity to argue for or against the injunction. The case had been assigned to Judge Joseph H. Hood, known among Lexington attorneys to be plainspoken on the bench—almost folksy—but fair and smart.

On July 5, 2005, Roger and Linda Thacker and several of the other Kentucky patients filed into the courthouse in downtown Lexington. They passed through the metal detector and took the elevator to the second floor and Judge Hood's courtroom. Given the building's nondescript exterior, its unexceptional hallways and the judge's own dressed-down demeanor on the bench, the room is surprisingly ornate. The ceiling is high and supported by a lattice of thick mahogany beams that stretch above tall, arched windows. At one end of the room towers the judge's bench. On the opposite wall, so that it is plain view of the judge as he looks over the courtroom, is a 15-foot-tall painting that depicts frontiersman Daniel Boone's arrival in Kentucky.

Hanging every dozen feet or so on the gray marble walls are the portraits of former judges. Below each is a plaque that gives the name of the judge, the years of his tenure, and the name of the president who appointed him. It was in this room that in 1949, Judge H. Church Ford ruled that the 14th Amendment to the U.S. Constitution required the University of Kentucky to admit African American students to its graduate schools. It was a landmark ruling at the time and surely surprised many who heard the verdict that day. The Thackers were hopeful that the day's hearing would yield a similarly surprising verdict. Amgen had won a favorable ruling from Judge Castel in New York, and the company clearly had the upper hand. Judge Hood wasn't bound by the New York district court's decision, but surely Amgen would cite it in their case, and it was possible that the judge simply would defer to it and deny the Kentucky patients in similar fashion.

Roger Thacker was in a wheelchair. Not only were his Parkinson's symptoms worsening, but his hip had been bothering him. Linda positioned Roger in the wheelchair in an inconspicuous spot near the back of the room. When Alan Milstein entered the courtroom, however, he told Roger to move closer to the front of the rows of mahogany benches. He would make a powerful visual aid.

Also in the room was Perry Cohen, executive director of the Parkinson's Pipeline Project, the nonprofit group that took up the

GDNF patients' fight early. Mr. Cohen had flown from Baltimore to witness the hearing. For years he had been advocating his vision of a research subject's bill of rights, a document that would serve as a model for how companies and research institutions should craft their own ethics policies regarding research subjects. He saw in the GDNF case an example of what can occur in the absence of a policy that gives patients an active role in the research process.

Judge Hood emerged just after 9:30 A.M., and the hearing got underway. Seated with Mr. Milstein at the plaintiff's table was Debra Doss, a veteran Lexington attorney who had done most of the actual filing for the case. Across the aisle sat the Amgen contingent, led again by Mr. Gately.

"I have looked over the papers," Judge Hood began. "I am fairly familiar with the facts of the case, Mr. Milstein. So we don't really need to go into a lot of the facts. We just need to know why you think your clients warrant a preliminary injunction."[43]

"Certainly, your honor," the lawyer responded. "You know, Amgen, in their papers, are trying to convince this court that the drug is unsafe and not effective. But that's not the issue for the court. The issue for the court . . ."

"Who makes that decision?" the judge ventured.

"That's the issue. Who makes the decision."

It was soon clear that Mr. Milstein's approach to the Kentucky hearing would be different. Rather than try to prove that GDNF worked, as he had done in New York, he instead argued that the Kentucky patients' informed consent documents gave the principal investigators sole authority to decide whether safety concerns outweighed any benefit. The Kentucky doctors universally supported reinstating the trials, and it should be their prerogative—not Amgen's—to determine whether the trials should continue, Mr. Milstein argued.

He conceded that the informed consent document *did* authorize the "funding agency" of the study to halt the trials for a variety of reasons, but the document didn't specify what this "funding agency" was. Mr. Milstein argued that the University of Kentucky was the funding agency, since the university's doctors and nurses had carried out the trials. Either that, he said, or Amgen intentionally left patients in the dark about its position as the "funding agency."

"It's one of two possibilities," he told the judge. "Either the University of Kentucky or perhaps some other government agency like the FDA is the agency, or Amgen didn't want to tell the plaintiffs, the subjects here, that it was retaining the right to terminate the study. Why would they do that? Well, when you have subjects with a horrible disease, and they are so desperate that they are agreeing to have holes drilled in their heads, pumps inserted in their stomachs, catheters taken from their stomach all the way up into the brain—such extraordinary measures which themselves are extremely risky—those subjects might not agree to be in such a study, if they thought that some corporation out on the West Coast, whose business [was to make] money, that they were the ones to decide the medical reason as to whether or not to continue the drug."

The argument placed Amgen's legal team in an awkward position. Either the defense would have to concede that the company was not the funding agency (and thus cast doubt on Amgen's authority to halt the trial) or Mr. Gately and his team would have to argue that Amgen was, in fact, the funding agency and would have to explain why the company had not been straightforward in identifying itself that way.

Next, Mr. Milstein tried to set the GDNF case apart from previous cases that involved patients seeking experimental drugs. He referred to several cases that Amgen had cited in its court filings, cases in which patients suffering from AIDS and other serious illnesses had sued for access to drugs despite a general consensus among doctors that the drugs were ineffective.

"No one would argue if a drug is not safe—if the principal investigators decide the drug is not safe or effective—that the plaintiffs should then still say, 'I am entitled to it, I want it, I think it works for me.' We are not going to—going to let the patients run the hospital.

"You know, all the cases that Amgen cites to the contrary, all those cases that were involved, you know, back in the early research of AIDS, for AIDS drugs, when you had researchers saying, 'This drug doesn't work,' but you had AIDS patients saying, 'I want it anyway . . .

"That's not what this case is about. This case is about a study in which Amgen has delegated the role of deciding whether the drug is safe and effective to the principal investigators of the University of Kentucky. Those principal investigators of the University of Kentucky say it works and it's safe."

Judge Hood changed the subject with a question: "But if it's not safe, who bears the fault? Do the principal investigators? Do the principal investigators stand up and say, 'My fault, my fault. My most grievous fault. You have developed these problems that we have seen . . .'"

"Well, your honor . . ."

". . . that 'it's my fault' or are they going to say, 'It's not my fault. It's Amgen's fault'? Who is going to get hit with the fault? Now, I have been around here for a long time doing this kind of work. And believe me, somebody is going to point the finger at somebody. Is Amgen going to be the one to have the finger pointed at them or the Kentucky doctors or the University of Kentucky hospital? Now I know there is a statement, there is an argument: 'Well, we can waive any liability.' Well, I have been here long enough to know that there are bright lawyers that can poke holes in any waiver that anybody has ever signed."

The judge's question got at the heart of what Amgen stood to lose by allowing access to GDNF. His implication was that if something went wrong, Amgen would be held accountable. No document, no waiver of liability could be drafted so as to guarantee 100 percent that some future judge or jury would not throw it out. The only completely safe route Amgen could take was the one it had chosen: no GDNF for anyone for any reason.

Be that as it may, Mr. Milstein said, such considerations shouldn't influence how the judge ruled on this particular case. "That can't be the reason why this court hesitates to issue the order that we have requested," he said to the judge. "That can't be the reason."

"Okay," replied the judge.

"I mean, if the court finds there is no agreement the way the court found in New York, which flies in the face of the document you have before you, that's one thing," Mr. Milstein said. "But if that's the reason, then that's the reason."

"All right, thank you," the judge said, putting an end to the discussion. "Mr. Gately?"

As he had done in New York, Mr. Gately rose and stood before the judge. Before he could begin, Judge Hood asked, "Now, why can't we give twenty-four months' worth of drugs to these people?"

Amgen's lawyer took the question in stride.

"Because it would be wrong on the contract documents here," he said. "The only contract Amgen entered into was a study contract with the University of Kentucky. And it would fly in the face of specific FDA regulations in the entire scheme for conducting the entire study.

"It also, perhaps most importantly, to get away from the law for a moment, would violate the first principle of the Hippocratic Oath.

It would violate the principle of 'do no harm.' Amgen has found this drug based on hard scientific data to present serious safety factors under those circumstances."

Judge Hood interjected: "Well, Mr. Milstein says that it doesn't —the contract doesn't allow Amgen to make that determination as opposed to the [contract] in New York," the judge said.

"And Mr. Milstein is my friend," replied Mr. Gately, "but I respectfully disagree with him factually and legally here, your honor."

Mr. Gately then spoke of how companies test their experimental drugs through independent researchers to avoid conflicts of interest. A sponsor like Amgen will contract with a research institution like the University of Kentucky to conduct the trial. The research institution functions as a buffer between the sponsor and the patients.

"The sponsors are not supposed to be involved with the clinical studies but are supposed to be back far enough away from the clinical subjects so that it has no involvement with them, and it only deals with the data on an objective basis, which is exactly what Amgen did here," Mr. Gately said. The only contract Amgen had signed was with the University of Kentucky, he argued, and the wording of that contract regarding Amgen's ability to stop the trials was clear: "This agreement may be terminated by Amgen immediately upon written notice."

The defense's argument in Kentucky was the same that it had been in New York: Amgen couldn't be held liable for breach of contract with the patients because there simply was no contract, and there was no grounds for a *promissory estoppel* claim because there was no promise.

Before he concluded the hearing, Judge Hood said a few words in closing.

"I understand the particular significance of this matter because of personal familiarity with the ravages of Parkinson's disease," he said. "So I appreciate the quality of arguments and the quality of the papers in this particular matter. It makes it a lot easier for me to make this decision, and I should have something out by the end of the week."

Roger Thacker's wheelchair was in the center of the room and directly in Judge Hood's line of sight. As the judge spoke, Roger tried to catch his eye. When the judge's eyes met his own, Roger pressed his palms together in front of his chest as if supplicating in prayer, and he slowly mouthed the word "please."

33 Discovery

Judge Hood denied the patients' request. His ruling came just three days after the hearing, on July 8, 2005. In his written opinion, he described why he believed the patients' lawsuit fell short, and he elaborated on his comment during the hearing that he had a "personal familiarity with the ravages of Parkinson's disease."

"Although the court personally understands the devastation Parkinson's brings to the lives of those who have the disease (my late father suffered from it) and the plaintiffs' immense desire for a cure, the public interest would not be furthered by ordering a clinical trial sponsor to provide unapproved and potentially dangerous drugs to clinical trial participants," Judge Hood wrote.

The appeals process would drag on for another year, but each higher court agreed with the lower courts' rulings. Eventually both the New York and the Kentucky lawsuits were dismissed. It became clear to the patients that they would have no recourse through the courts.

A remarkable thing occurred in July of 2005, the same month Judge Hood made his ruling. The doctors in Bristol had remained fairly quiet in the GDNF debate and unlike the other investigators from the North American trial sites had not participated in the lawsuits. In July, Dr. Gill and his associates at Frenchay published an article in the science journal *Nature Medicine* that seemed to offer the best evidence yet that the patients' improvements on GDNF were not simply imagined.[44]

In December of 2004, Henry Webb, the first of the five original patients in Bristol to receive GDNF, had died of an unrelated heart attack. His surviving family had agreed to allow the Frenchay doctors to perform an autopsy and examine his brain. Of the five men who volunteered in that first clinical trial, Henry was the only one who had GDNF pumped into just one side of his brain; the other four had pumps and catheters on both sides. Of the five, only his brain would allow the Frenchay scientists to compare the GDNF-treated side with the untreated one.

The title of the July 2005 article leaves little doubt about what the Bristol doctors found: "GDNF induces neuronal sprouting in human brain." When Henry Webb started the GDNF trials, his Parkinson's symptoms had been most severe on the left side of his body, indicating that the right side of his brain was most affected. Dr. Gill had implanted a catheter into Henry's right *putamen,* and for 43 months, Henry had received GDNF continuously at varying doses.

The autopsy revealed that after more than three years on GDNF, Henry had significantly more dopamine-producing neurons in the right *putamen* than in the left. The side of his brain that was once the most damaged by the disease now appeared to be the least scathed. In the tissue near where the catheter tip had been, there was a fivefold increase in dopamine fibers and neurons compared to the untreated left side.[45]

Perhaps most interesting was how the autopsy data matched Henry's motor scores during those 43 months. During the first two years of the study, the afflicted left side of Henry's body steadily improved. The right side remained as good as ever. At about 24 months, however, Henry began to notice that Parkinson's was overtaking the once-healthy right side of his body. What was once his "normal" half was becoming more and more afflicted, while his once-weaker side was steadily improving.

The courts had not addressed the question of whether GDNF worked. Both judges ruled that because there was no evidence of a contract between Amgen and the patients, there was no need for the court to decide whether the drug had made patients better. Had the courts considered the issue, Henry Webb's autopsy would have provided the most compelling evidence that GDNF did, in fact, cause once-shriveled brain cells to re-sprout and that the sprouting was accompanied by a general improvement in motor function. Even though it didn't help them much in court, the report did seem to validate at least one of the patients claims: that the improvements on GDNF were not simply the placebo effect but rather the result of a real and substantial change in the brain.

Unfortunately for the patients, proving to Amgen that GDNF worked was only half of the equation. The other half, the more critical half, was proving that the drug was safe. As the Vioxx case had shown, safety issues could quickly submarine an otherwise beneficial drug. The brain damage in the monkeys continued to be a major stumbling block. If Amgen, for whatever reason, was determined not to resume the trials, the brain damage provided strong support for their position. And if the company *were* interested in returning GDNF to the patients, the brain damage was a lingering issue that would need to be resolved.

In September of 2005, the CBS news program *60 Minutes* aired a report on the GDNF trials. Reporter Leslie Stahl had read in the *New York Time*s about the failed GDNF lawsuits and decided the patients' story was a good fit for the program. The Thackers, the Kaufmans, the Suthers and several other patients I spoke with said they had high hopes for what Ms. Stahl's report would achieve. After all, it was the top-rated news magazine program in the country. Perhaps the *60 Minutes* piece would accomplish what the lawsuits could not.

Amgen would not grant an interview for the story, but the company did release a statement. In it, Amgen stated that it would continue to withhold GDNF in order to protect the patients "against the possibility of drug-induced adverse effects."[46]

The program aired, and the profile of the GDNF debate was elevated to new heights, but for the patients, not much changed. Each scathing report seemed to solidify Amgen's resolve. The company steadfastly insisted that it had done the responsible thing in halting the trials and withholding the drug.

Throughout 2005 and into early 2006, the GDNF issue became an increasingly divisive one in the Parkinson's research community. In December of 2005, *Lancet Neurology,* a respected science journal, published an editorial titled "The hard way to a Bill of Rights." The editorial urged Amgen to allow compassionate use of GDNF and to analyze how the different catheter systems in each of the trials might have affected their outcomes. It also lauded the efforts of some patients to create a so-called research subject's bill of rights, a document that would guide companies and research institutions in the way they design and administer clinical trials. In closing, the editorial supported the patients' claim that GDNF should be returned.

> The patients in this case were willing to accept any risks when they agreed to participate in Amgen's study. However, none of them anticipated that those risks would include

> the termination of a potentially beneficial treatment, leaving them with no alternative therapy. It is understandable that these patients now ask for the respect, beneficence and justice that should guide clinical trials."

The editorial prompted a response[47] from Dr. Lang, Dr. Nutt, Dr. Wooten, Dr. Stacy, and other investigators who had supported Amgen's decision to halt the trials, which in turn prompted a response[48] from the Dr. Penn, Dr. Hutchinson, and the Kentucky doctors, who had remained critical of Amgen's decision. Strongly worded letters to the editor began to show up in other journals, written by scientists with no direct involvement in the GDNF trials.[49]

Such was the state of things when I first heard of GDNF.

34 Roger Thacker:

Twenty-one months after losing GDNF

I learned of GDNF when the story seemed to be arriving at its inevitable conclusion. The patients' numerous appeals to Amgen for compassionate use had been denied, and both civil lawsuits had dead-ended. Several of the stalwarts in Bristol and Kentucky who once had refused to have the pumps removed had reluctantly acquiesced. By the time I began visiting patients in their homes in the summer of 2006, only a handful still carried the bulky metal pumps inside.

In early June I traveled to Lexington, Kentucky to the home of Roger and Linda Thacker. They had offered me a room for the few days I was in town, and my first inclination was to decline, to keep the appropriate distance between myself and my subject matter. I reconsidered when I thought of how beneficial it could be to observe Roger Thacker in his own home at various times of the day and night.

I drove from the Lexington's Bluegrass Airport through the eastern edge of the city until I reached the state highway that would lead me south to the tiny community of Versailles. The highway snakes through the sloping green hills of country clubs and horse farms. The Thacker's home was a newer ranch-style rambler at the end of a gravel road. Fifty acres of fields surrounded the house, and at the perimeter of the fields dark pine trees lined the property like an enormous hedge surrounding an immense lawn. The fields were sectioned off by fences, but there was no livestock that I could see. The hay had grown high and looked ready for cutting.

Linda Thacker met me in the driveway, both to greet me and to protect me from the affections of Churchill, the family's massive grand Pyrenees. "You made it," she said warmly as she clutched Churchill's collar. Linda is of average height with graying hair, a youthful face, and expressive blue eyes. She led me into the modest but immaculate home with spotless hardwood floors and windows that let in plenty of natural light. When I walked in the door, I immediately smelled a minty odor. It was familiar, but I couldn't identify it. The smell wasn't overpowering, but it was noticeable.

Roger sat in the living room in a tall chair with a metal walker in front of him. Even seated he appeared tall and gaunt. He has a thin face, deep-set eyes and high, prominent cheekbones. It was a warm day, and he wore shorts and a white knit tank top. An open jar of Icy Hot was on a nearby table and the skin of his legs and upper arms were glistening from a recent application of the stuff. This was the familiar smell—the topical pain cream that I had seen used in athletic settings.

Roger's hair was white and wispy, and his hairline had receded so that I could easily spot a small lump on the crown of his head. I knew it was one end of a 1-mm catheter that plunged into his brain. Through it, Roger received GDNF for almost two years. Now it pumped only saline solution.

"I'm afraid I'm not 'on' and I'm not 'off' but somewhere in between," he said breathlessly.

Roger would later tell me that his father had been a very private man, who never spoke openly about his own medical condition. I sensed that, in addition to Parkinson's, Roger had inherited some of his father's private nature. Even in shorts and a tank-top and smeared with pain ointment, Roger projected an air of propriety and British reserve. He seemed uncomfortable holding himself out for the world to see and for journalists to probe with personal questions. In a let's-get-this-over-with kind of way, Roger asked if I would like to interview him immediately. But I said no, that there would be plenty of time during the next two days.

Then Linda directed me to the guest room. Like the rest of the house, it was immaculate. There were bookshelves built into one wall and I browsed the titles. There were many from prominent American conservatives and several religious titles. I learned that Linda is a devoutly religious woman. She was born into the Church of Jesus Christ of Latter-day Saints and remained an active Mormon throughout her life. Two sons from her first marriage volunteered as Mormon missionaries, and Linda speaks proudly of them and easily and about her beliefs.

Roger is much more reticent about his faith. He told me that he does believe in God, and he has contemplated how his experience with GDNF might fit into some greater plan. He had attended church with Linda many times over the years but, as of our meeting, had not converted to his wife's faith. Hoping that publicizing his own plight would help him to recover GDNF, he had sacrificed much of his precious privacy. His medical condition and his affected body became fodder for local and national media outlets, and perhaps that much was a necessary evil in order to recover GDNF. He said he felt there was little to be gained, however, in airing his religious beliefs. His personal disclosures only went as far as their utility.

During the first hour or so of my visit, Roger was close to immobile. Eventually he did rise to his full height of well over six feet, and, swinging and planting the metal walker with broad motions, retired to his bedroom. The small master bedroom was mostly filled with the large hospital-type bed that had knobs and buttons for adjusting the bed to its least-uncomfortable position. Near the bed was a small television and a VCR with movies stacked on top of and around it; mostly they were John Ford-era Westerns. A computer and printer sat on the nearby table. From it, Roger had sent several e-mails to me in the weeks leading up to my visit. (E-mail was the most effective way of communicating with the patients. Phone calls were hit-and-miss because some patients, including Roger, could not speak clearly during their "off" periods. E-mails they could answer at their leisure.)

Even when he was out of the living room, I could judge Roger's condition by how frequently he called on Linda for assistance—to adjust the bed, massage a sore muscle, smear on the Icy Hot, bring a glass of water, and so on. I would be speaking with Linda in the living room or kitchen, and Roger's accented voice would rise plaintiff from the other room: "Lin-*dah*?" She would stop mid-sentence and disappear down the hallway. Sometimes she would have scarcely returned when the cry would come again, "Lin-*dah*?"

I began to realize in my first hours with the Thackers that Parkinson's is a disease that afflicts in pairs. Patients with advanced-stage Parkinson's require a caregiver a lot of the time, and both lives are very much tied up in the disease. Relief for the patient is relief for the caregiver. According to the Thackers, GDNF had been both.

On the second day of my visit, Roger was a different man. He moved through the house in long, measured strides and with an apparent sense of urgency. He was "on," and he seemed determined to cram as much activity into those useful hours before his body shut off again. After breakfast, he announced that he would be cutting the hay that day. Linda voiced what seemed to me to be a token protest because it was in a tone that suggested she had no hope of changing his mind. She shook her head as Roger strode out the back door, his metal walker slung over his shoulder like a knapsack. I followed him out and watched him set the walker in the bed of a well-used pickup truck. He climbed in and then drove to the barn where his tractor was parked.

Roger has been a hard worker all his life. Linda said that during his tenure at the University of Kentucky, he would return from work in the evenings to give Linda a kiss, and then it was out the door to the fields for another three hours or so of work on the property. The active lifestyle he maintained previously must have made the disease all the more distressing. Like Steve Kaufman, the Chicago patient who had a passion for speed, Roger seemed to suffer more from Parkinson's because of the pace at which he had lived before it.

With Roger temporarily unavailable for an interview, I passed much of the morning sitting with Linda in her kitchen. She talked about her sons, two of whom lived near her in the Lexington area. She spoke of meeting Roger and coming to appreciate his eccentricities. At regular intervals during our conversation, the roar of an engine would rise outside the kitchen window, and I would look up in time to see Roger lumbering by on his tractor. First, he would pass from left to right, and a few minutes later he would appear farther away passing from right to left. The brief snapshots showed an active, able man. They revealed the man as he had been and perhaps as he still would be without the intrusion of Parkinson's.

Linda said Roger had had hip problems that plagued him during his time on GDNF. The problem was aggravated after GDNF was taken away, she said, when his Parkinson's symptoms began to resurface. An orthopedic doctor advised him to see a pain management doctor. The pain management doctor recommended an epidural, and as the doctor pushed the needle into Roger's spine, she hit a nerve that shot a fiery pain down Roger's leg and immobilized him for months. After the nerve healed, Roger finally underwent hip replacement surgery in the fall of 2005. As he recovered from that surgery, Linda said, he could finally gauge his Parkinson's symptoms without interference from the bad hip or the damaged nerve.

What Roger found, Linda said, was that he was a lot better off than when he started the GDNF trials. Eighteen months after losing the drug, he was much more mobile, his "on" times were significantly longer and more predictable, and he required far less of the pain relief ointment.

The engine roared again and I looked up and saw Roger speed by on his tractor. When I started my research, I knew my timing would put me at a disadvantage. I was coming at the story 18 months after the GDNF trials ended, so I would be writing from a limited perspective. Yet as I watched Roger motor by on his tractor, I realized my timing would provide me with at least one advantage: I would be able to observe the patients' condition after nearly two years without GDNF. If, as Amgen claimed, the patients' improvements had been the result of a prolonged "placebo effect," then surely the effect would have vanished after 18 months without GDNF. But if, after 18 months, patients continued to be improved over their pre-GDNF state, that would be some evidence that GDNF's benefit was not simply imagined or willed into existence. I was no clinician, but this experiment seemed to be one that a nonscientist could carry out.

During my visits with patients, I started to ask a simple question. After spending a day with the patient and the caregiver, I would ask both of them, "Prior to receiving GDNF, how would this day have gone differently for you, if at all?" I asked it first of Roger and Linda Thacker after spending two days in their home. Roger answered this way:

"Before receiving the product [GDNF], I could not have done the work I have—cutting the hay and the outside work. I didn't have the energy to do that sort of thing. And sometimes I would be working outside, or trying to work outside, and I would just freeze up, and I was far away from the house, so Linda couldn't hear me. I would just have to wait until I could move again or until Linda found me.

"Now that my leg and my hip are improved, I am just beginning to see how I am, to see what the drug did for me. And I believe there's been some regrowth there, I do. I am more active and mobile than before I got the drug."

Linda said, "Roger still goes 'off,' as you know, but now he's getting back on the tractor. GDNF definitely has maintained some of the improvement. Before GDNF, he had given up on the animals and some of the things he does now. Now he's talking about getting some ewes and other animals to take care of.

"He went to a meeting last Saturday. It was maybe three-and-a-half hours long. He would not have done that before GDNF. He could be walking across the room and freeze. He could be walking to shake someone's hand and freeze. Since GDNF, the freezing has not occurred."

This is not to say that Roger was active all or even most of the time. He passed much of the day, especially the afternoons, sitting in his chair or resting on his bed. He or Linda still would apply Icy Hot several times a day. Once he called me into his room to observe how the muscles of his leg had seized up. At his invitation, I pressed my finger against his calf muscle and found it tightly flexed, as if Roger were standing on his tip-toes. It remained that way for close to an hour as Roger winced.

Parkinson's, in other words, was still and increasingly a part of the Thackers' lives. Yet both said Roger was much better off than before GDNF. It was a compelling testimony, but I was skeptical because of Roger's previous hip problems. It was possible that even before he received GDNF, Roger's hip was slowing him down. Maybe it was the new hip, and not the effects of GDNF, that had improved his mobility during the past year. Of course, the new hip wouldn't account for the improvements he reportedly had while he was on GDNF (before the hip replacement), nor would it account for why Roger had stopped freezing. In any case, Roger's was just one patient's account and not scientifically conclusive on its own. I had made plans to visit patients in New York, Chicago, Indianapolis, and Bristol, England. I was curious to see how these patients were faring after more than a year without GDNF. But first, I would travel to California to interview an Amgen spokesman about the company's reasons for halting the trials.

35 Access to Amgen

I flew to Los Angeles in June of 2006 to meet David Krawitz, a director in Amgen's corporate communications department. It had taken several phone calls and e-mails to get this far. I had requested interviews with former members of Amgen's GDNF team and with Kevin Sharer, the CEO. Instead, I was referred to David, who said that before he arranged the interviews he first would like to meet me in person and provide some material that Amgen's legal staff would put together. We would meet at the bar of Casa Del Mar, a swank hotel on Santa Monica's beach with a pool and a restaurant that overlook the ocean.

I was disappointed to learn that David had joined Amgen less than six months earlier and that what he knew about GDNF he had learned after being hired. I had been hoping to speak with someone directly involved in the trials, but I did recognize the opportunity to get a foot in Amgen's door. I knew David would be sizing me up to decide whether Amgen should grant the other interviews I requested. He was the GDNF gatekeeper, and without his blessing I almost certainly would not have access to anyone else at the company.

I walked into the lobby of Casa Del Mar at 5 P.M. and scanned the lounge area. I found David as he had described over the phone, sitting by a low table in the lounge with four enormous three-ring binders stacked on the table in front of him.

A tall, stocky man with dark but graying curly hair, David is a public affairs veteran who worked in several staff positions in the U.S. Senate for 16 years before moving to Los Angeles in 2001 to join a global public relations firm. Amgen hired him in February 2006 as its senior director of global brand management and product communications. Among his many responsibilities, he had been assigned to deal with inquiries about the GDNF trials.

He invited me to ask questions about GDNF, and though he wouldn't be able to answer them on the spot he would get them to the people who could. The tone of the conversation was good-natured. David asked that I not record our interview, so I can't reproduce it here, but we spoke at length about Amgen, the company's mission and its priorities. David stressed that while other drug companies develop treatment for hair loss and erectile dysfunction, Amgen targets life-threatening diseases such as cancer and kidney disease. Its scientists are driven to develop new treatments to relieve human suffering. He said people work at Amgen not for the paycheck but because they care about patients and want to help sick people get better. And he was adamant that GDNF had not been shelved due to financial concerns. He referred to several products that the company was developing that benefit a relatively small group of patients worldwide.

I knew it was David's job to cast Amgen in this light. He was director of brand management, and this was the brand he hoped to put forward: Amgen as the biotech company that cares about patients, the company whose employees work tirelessly in pursuit of medical breakthroughs, not to make themselves rich or to satisfy shareholders, but simply to relieve human suffering.

After talking in the lounge for about an hour, he asked if I would like to have dinner at the hotel's restaurant. The restaurant is called Oceanfront and is well named. Our table overlooked Santa Monica's well-groomed beach, its lapping waves, and a low-hanging sun in the west. From my seat, I could see the Ferris wheel circling on Santa Monica pier less than a mile to the north. I took the dinner offer as a good sign. David could have ended the interview in the lounge, but he didn't. Once we moved to the restaurant, our conversation turned to our families, to David's recent vacation, and so on. Before the end of the meal, David had told me he would do what he could to arrange the interviews with Kevin Sharer and the others. He said he preferred a policy of transparency, and he said he sensed that I was interested in getting at the truth.

After dinner, he handed over the hefty binders, one by one. He said they contained all the legal filings from both of the lawsuits that GDNF patients filed against Amgen. It was public information, all of it available online through a federal court records search, but I appreciated that Amgen's legal team had compiled the documents. David said he would be in touch with the answers to my questions and about the status of the interviews. We exchanged business cards and parted.

36 Bob Suthers: Twenty-one months after losing GDNF

I traveled to New York City that same month to interview Bob and Elaine Suthers. I took the Long Island Railroad to Huntington Station on an overcast day. I had arranged to stay with a friend in the city while I was in town, and I would have only one afternoon to spend with the Suthers.

Bob and Elaine lived in Greenlawn within one mile of where Bob grew up. Elaine picked me up at Huntington Station just after noon and drove the few minutes to their home. I recognized the one-story white house from the recorded *60 Minutes* report I had watched many times. The report began with Bob leaving his front door and taking dozens of tiny, faltering steps across his driveway to retrieve a newspaper. When I walked in the door, Bob was seated in a recliner. He offered his hand and said what must have been the first thing that came into his mind.

"You are a lot younger than I expected," he said. "You look like the boys my daughter brings home."

I smiled and nodded. Bob and I had spoken briefly over the phone. He must have imagined a more veteran journalist on the other end of the line. Elaine would later explain that Bob's stroke stripped him of many inhibitions, resulting in some awkward and comical situations after Bob would blurt out the first thing that came to his mind.

For more than two years after losing GDNF, Bob had written regular letters to Amgen CEO Kevin Sharer. Bob doubted the envelopes would ever be opened, but he wrote them anyway, and as time passed, their tone became more and more bitter. In one letter that Bob wrote in mid-2006, he spoke of his own experience in the military, and in an off-hand way he wrote that Mr. Sharer probably wouldn't know anything about the honor and commitment military service requires. Several days later, Elaine was sitting in the family's living room with Bob when the phone rang. Bob answered the phone, and Elaine was stunned when Bob practically shouted into the phone, "You are an evil man!"

Elaine managed to pry away the phone and beg pardon of the man, who, to her great surprise, was in fact Kevin Sharer. He had called to set the record straight. Contrary to what Bob had implied in his letter, Mr. Sharer had a long and distinguished military career. He had attended the U.S. Naval Academy and had served in the Navy from 1970 to 1978. After getting over her initial surprise to find Amgen's CEO on the line, Elaine apologized for Bob's outburst. Ever since the stroke, she explained to me, he hadn't been himself.

I appreciated Bob's candor. His thoughts and feelings came through unfiltered. Elaine had made some sandwiches, and as we ate Bob spoke openly about his life in the monastery, his reasons for leaving and the years since then. He spoke of these subjects with obvious fondness, particularly when speaking of his three daughters.

His mood darkened when GDNF came up. Bob's initial frustration at losing the drug had been compounded with each unanswered letter. He became emotional as he spoke and he shed tears, which seemed to make him all the more frustrated. As Bob fought to regain composure, Elaine explained that one symptom of Parkinson's is that patients may become overly emotional. Bob nodded.

"Sometimes I will be talking and I will start crying and I have no idea why," he said, through tears. "I don't want to; it just happens sometimes."

The question of how Bob fared now compared to his pre-GDNF state was a tricky one because of the stroke that occurred at his first surgery. The stroke complicated the before-and-after comparison. Physically, the stroke had not affected him in a lasting way, but it had damaged him cognitively. During the first few weeks after it occurred, Bob was often disoriented and had trouble remembering names and faces. He eventually recovered most of what he had lost, but neurologists said his executive function, a term psychologists use to describe a theoretical command center that controls other cognitive processes, remained impaired.

In spite of this impairment, Bob said he experienced both physical and cognitive improvements on GDNF, relative to his pre-GDNF state. After six months on the saline placebo, Bob had received the drug for five months. That's when he successfully took the subway to the clinic downtown for his monthly visit, and his mask disappeared.

"When I learned they cancelled the trial, I was furious, immediately furious," he said. "I thought I would be going downhill right away. I thought the improvements were going to disappear within days, but it wasn't like that."

Elaine said that contrary to what they both feared, Bob actually continued to improve in the months after the trial ended. Only recently, she said, had she seen his progress peak and then slowly reverse.

"I think we had a plateau a few months ago. I've noticed that he is starting to slow down a little. But I don't think he's back to where he was before the GDNF," she said.

Amgen did not release individual patient data for the phase II trial, so Bob's motor scores before and after GDNF were never made public. What is known is that the 34 patients' average improvement fell short of the 25 percent increase Amgen had anticipated. Bob's neurologist, Dr. Hutchinson, was immediately skeptical of the company's analysis of the data. He had seen noticeable improvements in all three of his patients, all of whom had been in the placebo group of the study but then received GDNF for five months after the study ended.

In early 2003, when Amgen's scientists and the investigators were designing the phase II study, they anticipated a certain amount of "noise" in the data, irregularities caused by imperfect motor score assessments. They knew that because of the subjective nature of the Unified Parkinson's Disease Ratings Scale, where nurses observe patients as they complete various physical tasks, the patient population would need to be large enough to account for the variability in the assessments. Based on the noise that had been observed in the Bristol trial, the planners of the phase II trial assumed there would be a standard deviation of 20 percent. In reality, Hutchinson learned, the actual standard deviation had been closer to 25 percent. One of the study designers' key assumptions was off by a fairly significant margin. Hutchinson suspected that because of this, the study had been underpowered, that it included too few patients to draw definite conclusions. Yet, when Dr. Lang and several of the other investigators published the formal report on the study in March of 2006, they concluded that GDNF delivered via pump had not been effective: "We can rule out with good power a large beneficial clinical effect."[50]

Hutchinson did his own analysis of Amgen's data and asked a few independent statisticians to do the same. In July of 2006, Hutchinson and two biostatisticians published an article in the *Journal of Neuroscience Methods* that refuted the conclusion of Lang and the others. Hutchinson's co-authors were Susan Gurney, from Columbia University's School of Public Health, and Roger Newson, from the Heart and Lung Institute from Imperial College, London. Their article pointed to Amgen's failed phase II trial as an example of what can go wrong when scientists are overly cautious in concluding that a given treatment is effective. Researchers are too concerned about committing type I error (concluding that an ineffective treatment is effective) that they too often err in the opposite direction and commit type II error (concluding a good treatment is useless), the article stated.

"For the clinical investigator, a type I error risks the stigma of amateurish enthusiasm. If an error is to be made, a type II at least maintains the appearance of erring on the side of fastidiousness and caution."

Hutchinson and the co-authors had done two statistical tests, the "t-test" and the "rank-based Somers' D." They found that because of the greater-than-anticipated amount of statistical noise, the study was too small to conclude, as Lang and the others had, that a large clinical benefit from GDNF could be ruled out. Hutchinson's article stated that "the standard deviation of the . . . data turned out to be considerably higher than had been anticipated in the power analysis performed prior to the study.

"In order to determine what impact, if any, this had on the conclusions that could be drawn, the actual data were analyzed by means of both the t-test and the rank-based Somers' D. *The study was found to be underpowered and thus incapable of ruling out a large effect of GDNF on Parkinson disease. It therefore does not contradict the large effects seen in previous open-label studies*" (emphasis added).[51]

Hutchinson wasn't necessarily arguing that GDNF worked, only that the phase II study was too weak to conclude that it did not. In deciding to halt the trials, Amgen had assumed a benefit of zero from GDNF, based on the failed phase II study. Dr. Hutchinson's analysis challenged that assumption.

By the time Hutchinson published his article, however, nearly two years had passed since the patients lost GDNF. All but a handful had had their titanium-encased pumps removed, and many had received DBS instead. Bob Suthers was among the few holdouts who continued to hang on to a hope that he would recover GDNF. I could see the pumps bulging from beneath his T-shirt. Bob agreed with Elaine that he had not yet slid back to his pre-GDNF state, but he said there was no doubt that he was sliding.

"Before, my medication was cut in half, I could read the newspaper in the morning. Now, I can't concentrate more than half an hour." Elaine chimed in that Bob's ability to walk and to write had declined recently. Bob agreed, though he added that before GDNF he couldn't walk or write much at all, and he couldn't read much of the paper. That he could do these things now was an improvement.

Like Roger Thacker, Bob believed that even after more than one year without GDNF, he was still in better shape than before he got the drug. It was impossible for me to verify in an objective way whether that were true because, after Amgen cancelled the trials, the company stopped doing the monthly motor score assessments. Even if Amgen had continued to assess the patients, the company probably would not have made the data public. Still, the testimony of Roger Thacker, Bob Suthers and many of their family members was that both men were in better condition 21 months after losing GDNF than they were before they began the GDNF trials.

37 Doors of the Kingdom

Several weeks passed after my meeting with David Krawitz in Santa Monica, and we corresponded by telephone and e-mail. Finally David told me that, despite his best efforts to schedule the interviews I had asked for, Amgen's executives had decided against them. David said that the Amgen employees who were involved in the GDNF trial had suffered a great deal of emotional stress in the wake of the cancelled trials. These were people who had devoted a large portion of their professional lives to the development of GDNF, and they wanted to see it succeed as much as anyone, he said. They were anxious to put the whole affair behind them and get back to the business of finding new treatments. David said that he was sorry, but there was nothing he could do.

"If it were up to me, I would open the doors to the kingdom," he told me over the phone. "But it's not up to me."

David did get back to me with the answers to the 10 questions he had jotted down during our meeting. They were similar to the company's previous public statements, and they added little that was new. For example, one of my questions asked why Amgen had denied compassionate use of GDNF to the patients who already had received it, even though the FDA gave the green light. In response, Amgen stated, "Amgen feels it would be unacceptable to provide a drug to patients with no proven benefit and alarming safety concerns. In addition, an alternative approved therapy, deep brain stimulation, was available."

My efforts to speak with the investigators who had supported Amgen's decision to halt the trial were equally fruitless. I made numerous phone calls to the offices of Dr. John Nutt in Oregon and Dr. Frederick Wooten in Virginia. I also sent e-mails, asking for any comment, any information that would help me to tell the GDNF story. None of these messages were returned. Dr. Tony Lang from Toronto, who took the lead of Amgen's phase II trial, did return a phone call, but only to tell me that he preferred not to comment on the issue. Only Dr. Mark Stacy, the lead investigator at Duke in North Carolina, spoke to me at length about his reasons for supporting Amgen. He said he had no regrets about withdrawing GDNF from his patients because he believed it was not doing anything for them.

The other investigators would say nothing. Like Amgen, they seemed ready to move on.

38 Steve Kaufamn: Twenty-two months after losing GDNF

I traveled to Chicago in July of 2006 to interview Steve and Maggie Kaufman. The Kaufmans had invited me to stay in their home during the few days I was in town, and I accepted their invitation. I had spoken with Steve several times at the World Parkinson's Congress in Washington D.C., but I wanted to see how he passed the day at home.

The suburb of Algonquin in July is green and peaceful. The Kaufman's house is a tidy tri-level with a well-groomed yard and an asphalt driveway. Both Steve and Maggie work in the greater Chicago area. They eat out once or twice a week, and during my first evening with them, they took me to one of their favorite spots. It was a family restaurant called Nick's Pizza & Pub, a place that is famous for its unique atmosphere.

Steve drove us to Nick's in his black Pontiac Grand Am. We waited for about 10 minutes to be seated and snacked on peanuts in the waiting area. As is the custom at Nick's, we tossed the shells onto the floor, adding them to the carpet of shells that was already there. Steve's arm shook slightly as we ordered our pizzas, and his head was in a subtle but constant side-to-side motion, a side effect of the pills he was taking.

During the meal, Steve and Maggie told me about a cabin they were building in northern Wisconsin and about how much they liked the people up there. Maybe they would live there after retiring, they said. Steve had so many good childhood memories from the area, and Steve and Maggie through their visits had created many more good memories together.

After the meal, I asked the Kaufmans, "How would this night have been different before GDNF, if at all?"

Maggie said, "Well for one thing, the people at the other tables would have been staring at Steve and pointing. Now I don't think anybody really notices. I didn't see people looking."

"That's true," Steve said, nodding. "People would stare."

I asked Steve , "And what about driving? Would you have driven us here tonight?"

"Oh yeah, I could still drive before the GDNF," he assured me. Maggie looked across the table at Steve and then looked at me.

"He could drive," she said. "But I don't know if he should have been driving. He used to drive with one thumb on the steering wheel between his knees. He used to drive to work like that, and I used to get really nervous."

"Yeah, it was getting pretty bad," Steve admitted.

One notable difference between Steve Kaufman and the other two patients I had visited was his age. Steve was 49 years old when he started on GDNF, more than 10 years younger than Roger Thacker or Bob Suthers had been. He was one of the youngest patients to receive GDNF in any of the three pump-and-catheter trials. Some of the doctors speculated that Steve's relatively young age might account for his particularly dramatic improvements—and for why the improvements apparently persisted. Perhaps his younger brain cells were more easily revived.

There were still moments when Parkinson's made normal living impossible. Twice during our interviews in his home, Steve's right arm began to shake and he excused himself, explaining that the Sinemet had worn off and that there would be a delay of about half an hour before the new dose kicked in. During that half hour Steve stayed in his bedroom, out of sight. He would emerge 20 minutes later with only minor tremor in his arms and the slight shaking of his head. Steve seemed to be managing the disease quite effectively with his medication, which contrasted sharply with this description he gave of his pre-GDNF self, beginning with the moment he first noticed his Parkinson's symptoms: "Maggie had thrown a 40th birthday party for me, and it was about two in the morning. I noticed the little finger starting to twitch on my left hand. I thought, 'Ugh, I must be drinking too much.' About four o'clock in the morning we finally decided to end the party. I got up the next day and my finger was still twitching. I thought, 'Oh no, this is not good.'

"In December, Maggie rubbed my back because I was lifting weights. She felt a tremor in my shoulder blade. She was concerned about the tremors because my father had Parkinson's, also. She wanted to make sure I didn't have it.

"I went to the general practitioner. He examined me and said, 'You're too young to have Parkinson's.' He prescribed muscle relaxers, and when those didn't work, I went back two weeks later. He said, 'I'm going to have you see a neurologist.' "The neurologist in less than five minutes told me I had Parkinson's."

"For the first five years, I was able to hide it. I did the old Michael J. Fox trick—just put my hands in my pockets. When Michael J. Fox finally announced he had Parkinson's, it wasn't too much thereafter that people started asking me, 'Do you have Parkinson's Disease?' I figured I had to come clean because they're going to suspect anyhow. I came out and told them yes, I did have Parkinson's.

"At that time, I was the warehouse manager, and I told my boss. He was shocked. He asked me what the outcome of it was. I said, 'Right now it's treatable, but there's no cure. If you're asking me how bad can it get in the very near future, I don't know. Every patient is different.'

"Unfortunately, shortly thereafter, I took a nosedive—I started going downhill really quick. My boss said, 'I've got to make a real difficult decision. Either I have to offer you a different position or you'll have to leave the company. I can't have this department running in a different condition than what I'm accustomed to.'

"People started to become more and more aware about it. In about the eighth year, my neurologist told me, 'I can't give you more drugs. You're just about maxed out. I think you should go see another neurologist who's a specialist in this and talk to him about having a deep brain stimulator put in.'

"At that point, I was rapidly going downhill. Maggie tried to get me to go out for walks. I could only go about half a block. My legs would start buckling. The ankles would give out. She actually held on to my belt in the back to keep me from falling down, like a support.

"I said, 'Okay.'"

Steve had joined the trials because he had "maxed out" on Sinemet and his other medication. They no longer provided relief at any dose. That he could now subdue his symptoms with the same drugs was significant. It suggested that something in Steve's brain had changed. And, nearly two years later, the change had remained.

Shortly after Steve lost GNDF, he was interviewed by a reporter from the *New York Times*. I had read the *Times* article before I traveled to Chicago, and it came to mind as I observed Steve go about his day:

> With his condition deteriorating from Parkinson's disease last year, Steve Kaufman gave up making improvements to his home in Algonquin, Ill. "I couldn't even hold a nail stable," he recalled.
>
> Earlier this year, after taking an experimental drug in a clinical trial, Mr. Kaufman built new kitchen cabinets and an outdoor deck. He was so steady he could walk across a narrow piece of lumber like an Olympic gymnast on the balance beam.
>
> The drug, however, is no longer available to Mr. Kaufman or the other Parkinson's patients in clinical trials. [. . .]
>
> Amgen's move has provoked an outcry from patients who say the company is robbing them of their only hope. "It's almost the same thing as a diabetic losing their insulin," said Mr. Kaufman, who is 50 and has had Parkinson's for 10 years.[52]

When Amgen halted the trials, some demanded an explanation of how patients like Steve could show such improvements if the drug were ineffective, as Amgen had concluded that it was. Amgen's answer, and the explanation of Dr. Lang from Toronto, was that any *perceived* improvements were probably the result of a prolonged placebo effect.[53]

The placebo effect typically occurs when a patient expects that a treatment will be effective. The anticipation of benefit, even a subconscious one, is what produces the effect. It was clear from the distress that Steve expressed to the *New York Times*, however, that he believed he would suffer a great deal without the drug—as a diabetic might suffer without insulin. One might reasonably expect that any placebo effect Steve experienced while on the drug would quickly fade once GDNF was withdrawn and his expectations of it vanished. Yet Steve's improvements had apparently persisted despite his fears that they would not.

It was during my days with Steve Kaufman that I began to doubt seriously that the placebo effect could explain the patients' improvements. Twenty-one months after losing GDNF, the man who previously could not hold a nail stable was holding down a full-time job at a distribution center—and coolly navigating Chicago's stop-and-go traffic to get to and from it. He and Maggie also took regular trips to their property in northern Wisconsin and were just finishing a major construction project there, a cascading wooden staircase that would give them easy access to the lake that borders their plot of land. He could stand and walk for hours at a time without Maggie's hand on his belt.

In one of my interviews with her, Maggie said, "If Steve was in this good of shape when the trial started, they probably wouldn't have let him join." It was an interesting thought. The trial had been designed for advanced-stage patients. Steve's relatively good condition now very well might have disqualified him.

But while Steve's disease seemed to have reversed while he was on GDNF, his father's Parkinson's advanced at its normal, agonizing rate. In the summer of 2005, Steve visited his father in an assisted-living center in greater Chicago. He described the emotional visit and what transpired over the following weeks this way:

> One day we went to the nursing home and he wasn't there. Our first thought was, "Oh my God, he's passed away." And then we went to the nurse's station and they said, "Oh no, he's at the hospital on the North Shore." And I had never heard of this hospital. And I said, "What's he doing there?"

And they said, "They're doing surgery on him." And I go, "Surgery for what?" And the nurse said, ""You've got to talk to the doctor," so we call the doctor and the doctor says, "Well, we're closing off his bedsores."

I go, "Bedsores? What bedsores?" All the time that my brother and sister-in-law were taking care of him, he never once had a bedsore. And when they got to the point where they couldn't take care of him anymore and they took him to the nursing home, he started getting bedsores.

It got so bad that he got gangrene. The gangrene is what's the official cause of death, the infection. But he just suffered a horrible, horrible death. When he passed away, he was in a semi-fetal position—a lot of pain, a lot of pain. They had him on mega-doses of morphine and he was still in pain.

I remember the week before he passed away I went to see him. I was talking to him and I could see he was so upset. He said, "What are you doing here?" And I could hear him because I put my ear to his lips, and I could barely hear him saying that. I told him, "I've come to see you." And he says, "I don't want you seeing my like this." I said, "Well, I'm here, so deal with it." And he says, "You know, you're being a stubborn kraut," and I say, "Well, I learned it from a good teacher."

At that point, he really slipped away from us pretty quick. My brother went in to see him that morning and then came back to see him in the afternoon. But by that time, he had lost—he had left us. That was it.

Losing his father made Steve even more determined to regain access to GDNF. One of his main motivations for joining the trial had been to advance science toward a cure, maybe in time to do something for his father, who seemed to diminish by the day. It seemed to him a cruel irony that the closest thing he ever found to a cure—something that might have helped his dad and thousands of others—was being kept out of reach.

39 Martha Bohn

On one of the days that I was in Chicago, I drove downtown to interview a woman that I hoped would shed more light on why the GDNF trials had been halted. Martha Bohn was now a neurologist at Northwestern University Medical School who directed the neurobiology program at the Children's Memorial Research Center. It was Bohn who, along with Dave Schubert from the Salk Institute, identified the B49 cell line as a promising place to look for GDNF. Synergen somehow acquired the B49 cell line in the early 1990s and from it extracted GDNF. Synergen's scientists had decided that the best way to deliver GDNF would be to pump it directly into the brain. Dr. Bohn disagreed. She saw promise in the emerging field of gene therapy.

In gene therapy, scientists try to alter the genetic code of a person's cells or tissue, usually by engineering a virus to deliver new genetic material into existing cells. The hope is that the new genetic material will change the nature of the cell. Gene therapy is most commonly used to replace an "abnormal," disease-causing gene with a "normal" one. Thus the most common targets for gene therapy studies are diseases caused by single-gene defects, such as cystic fibrosis or sickle cell anemia.

In the case of GDNF, the viruses would be engineered to deliver a DNA sequence that, once incorporated by the host cell, would cause the cell to begin churning out GDNF on its own. In essence, it would create GDNF factories out of patients' existing neurons. Doctors would inject the reengineered virus into the middle brain, and the virus would do the rest. There would be no pumps, no tubes under the skin and no monthly refilling.

At the time that Bohn began exploring the gene therapy option for GDNF, however, the science was still in its infancy and riddled with problems. One difficulty was the chore of convincing patients and regulators to allow the patients to be injected with viruses that by their nature are unpredictable and difficult to control. Another problem was finding a way to limit how far the virus will spread into surrounding cells—creating an "off" switch for the virus to stop its march.

At that point, the scientists at Synergen and Dr. Bohn, therefore, began to pursue divergent paths to GDNF delivery. The company experimented with various ways of infusing man-made GDNF into the brain, and Dr. Bohn began to explore the possibilities of gene therapy. After Amgen acquired Synergen in 1994, the company continued in Synergen's vein. By 1999 Amgen's own research of infusion had dead-ended and GDNF was placed on a back burner. Then Dr. Gill from Bristol and the doctors from Kentucky approached the company with their pump-and-catheter idea.

GDNF delivery research was at another crossroads. Gene therapy had made some progress during the 1990s, and several gene therapy clinical trials had received FDA approval. Amgen might have opted to change gears and delve into gene therapy delivery at that time. However, in 1999, gene therapy suffered a major setback with the death of Jesse Gelsinger, the young man whose family Alan Milstein had represented before taking up the GDNF case. Recall that the 18-year-old died from multiple organ failures four days after starting the treatment at the University of Pennsylvania, and his death was believed to have been caused by a severe immune response to the therapy. To critics of gene therapy, Gelsinger's death underscored how immature the field still was. And in the 1999 to 2000 period, his death would have provided Amgen with a very good reason to avoid gene therapy delivery of GDNF.

Amgen ultimately elected to continue developing the infusion delivery method and gave the green light to Dr. Gill in Bristol for his pump-and-catheter trial in 2001. Meanwhile, Dr. Bohn continued to develop the gene therapy delivery method. She and her team at the Children's Memorial Research Center tested the therapy in rats and published several studies on their successes between 2000 and 2003.

Dr. Bohn has happy, smiling eyes and an easygoing demeanor that belies her fierce intelligence. She had asked that I invite Steve Kaufman to the interview in her office. She had read about Steve's improvements in the *New York Times* and elsewhere, and as someone who followed the GDNF controversy closely she wanted to meet him in person. Both Steve and Maggie were reluctant at first; they said they were concerned that Dr. Bohn might try to recruit them for another clinical trial. I told Steve that Dr. Bohn dealt only in rats, and then he said he would like to come along.

Dr. Bohn spoke of the GDNF trials in a tired, exasperated tone. She said that she, her graduate student, Jurgen Engele, and the Salk Institute's Dave Schubert had been on the verge of finding GDNF back in 1991. They had been looking for funding when Synergen announced that it had discovered the elusive neurotrophic factor. Dr. Bohn said things would have turned out much differently if she, rather than a private company, had patented the protein.

"I'd let everyone have it," she said. "It's very frustrating to see a company have such a tight grip on a protein like GDNF."

Dr. Bohn also told me something about Amgen's that I had not heard before. She said that in early 2004, Amgen approached her and some of her colleagues unexpectedly. Amgen's scientists were finally interested in developing a gene therapy delivery of GDNF, and they asked if Dr. Bohn and the others would be willing to collaborate with the company. This began a two-year professional relationship between Amgen and a consortium of neurologists from various academic research institutions that had adopted the name of Parkinson's Disease Gene Therapy Study Group. A neurologist named Howard Federoff at the University of Rochester in New York headed the Amgen initiative and was the consortium's liaison with the company. Federoff later told me that between February of 2004 and February of 2006 he made five or six visits to Thousand Oaks to meet with Amgen officials. Amgen's goal, he said, was to "hammer out a logical gene therapy product" using GDNF to treat Parkinson's.

"We agreed with Amgen that we would pursue this in a way that would be at first a small-scale phase I clinical trial that would look at safety and tolerability," Dr. Federoff said. In other words, even before Amgen received the negative results from its phase II pump-and-catheter trial, the company already was looking to delve into gene therapy delivery. And even after Amgen halted the pump-and-catheter trials, in the fall of 2004, and while the patients' lawsuits came and went, the company continued to pursue a gene therapy clinical trial. Then in late February of 2006, Dr. Federoff's contact at Amgen informed him quite abruptly that the company was no longer interested in collaborating with the Parkinson's Gene Therapy Study Group. After two years of regular visits and, by Dr. Federoff's estimation, hundreds of hours of work to design a phase I clinical trial for gene therapy delivery of GDNF, Amgen walked away.

This development left Dr. Bohn, Dr. Federoff, and their other colleagues in the group to speculate why the company would withdraw so abruptly. Dr. Federoff said Amgen's officials repeatedly expressed concern about who would have control of the data and about how much federal funding would be used in developing their product. Federal law allows the government to force a company to provide a drug if the company isn't making a good-faith effort to bring the drug to market, but only if the drug was developed with significant federal funding. The government has never exercised these so-called "march-in rights," but the law grants to the National Institutes of Health the authority to do so. As one might imagine, major pharmaceutical companies are extremely resistant to the exercise of these march-in rights. By partnering with the Parkinson's Gene Therapy Study Group, Amgen would be benefiting from a decade of research, much of it federally funded, in the gene therapy field. Dr. Federoff said he suspected that Amgen had decided not to expose itself to the risk of government interference and so had walked.

Dr. Bohn said she believed Amgen might have decided to develop its own gene therapy product in house. She said that after two years of meeting with the study group, Amgen's scientists might have decided they had learned enough.

"I think Amgen is actually thinking of doing GDNF gene therapy in an internal program," she said. "I think they got the information they needed from us, and they're going ahead and doing it. But I still don't know if they can do it right. They haven't done anything else right." Amgen would not comment on its plans for a gene therapy product.

When I asked her about her plans for the future, Dr. Bohn's mood brightened considerably. Gene therapy, she said, had started to shake the stigma that attached to it after Jesse Gelsinger's death. Companies like Amgen were beginning to glimpse gene therapy's potential to simplify protein delivery, and the FDA was finally approving clinical trials for gene therapy treatments in the brain.

"When we started, the whole field was not ready for that idea. It was very hard to get a grant. There were comments made, 'Oh, gene therapy will never be used in humans, and it definitely will never be used in the brain.' Now there are over 700 gene therapy protocols in the clinic and for the brain there are about six, I think. So, it's happening. It just took a long time for the science community to catch up to that idea. And it hasn't happened for GDNF gene therapy yet, but it's going to."

Dr Bohn said that she and Dr. Federoff and a neurosurgeon named Krys Bankiewicz from the University of California, San Francisco, planned to move forward with a clinical trial for gene therapy delivery of GNDF. When I asked if Amgen might object to the research, Dr. Bohn explained that Amgen would likely allow the product to progress through the several phases of clinical trials before claiming patent infringement or some other intellectual property violation.

"If you do a gene therapy trial in phase I, phase II, and phase III and everything works, then you have a product and that's when you start making money on it. That's where Amgen may have a problem. It's not clear what would happen at that point."

After our interview Dr. Bohn led me and Steve on a tour of her labs, where graduate students in white lab coats peered through safety goggles into test tubes and microscopes. They were young—about my own age—and appeared very focused. I wondered what kind of medical breakthroughs they would witness during their lifetime. I was beginning to get a sense of how long the road to a useful treatment really is. If one of those test tubes contained a breakthrough for Parkinson's, how old would those students be when it finally reached the market? Or would it reach the market at all?

On the ride back to Algonquin, Steve thanked me for taking him with me to meet Dr. Bohn. "It's good to know that people are still trying to do something with this drug," he said. "It really does work."

40 Case #6: Bob Cameron

The drive from Chicago to Indianapolis takes about three hours, and I used most of it to try to decide what to say to a widow who lost her husband to Parkinson's one month before. I had learned about Sherry Cameron just a week before the Chicago trip. Her husband Bob had been a GDNF patient at the trial site at the University of Chicago.

Back in early 2003, Sherry was losing Bob to Parkinson's, and she searched the Internet for anything that might do more for him than his medication. The searching led her to promising news reports about GDNF. She read about the successful trials in Bristol and Kentucky, and she learned that there was also a new, larger trial starting up at several cities around the world. She came across the name of Dr. Michael Hutchinson, and she contacted him at NYU. He told Sherry that a phase II trial of GDNF had just got underway; it really wasn't feasible for Bob to travel to the trial site at NYU, but Dr. Hutchinson told her that doctors at the University of Chicago were overseeing one of the sites. She called Dr. Richard Penn in Chicago and asked if Bob could enroll immediately. Dr. Penn was reluctant at first because of the distance, but Sherry said she and Bob were willing to make the three-hour trip. The advanced stage of Bob's disease qualified him for the trial, and he enrolled.

Each month, Bob and Sherry would drive the three hours to the University of Chicago Medical Center to have Bob's pumps refilled. It happened like that for six months with no significant change in Bob's condition. After the six-month study, in early 2004, Bob and Sherry learned that Bob had not been receiving the drug—he had been randomly assigned to the placebo arm of the trial—but Bob was given the option to sign on to a two-year follow-up study in which he would receive GDNF. He got his first dose in July of 2004 and a second dose in August. Amgen halted the trials the month after that.

When I knocked, Sherry opened the door to the house, which sat at the edge of a golf course in an affluent suburb called Fishers, just northeast of Indianapolis. She wasn't the sullen, red-eyed woman I was expecting. She showed me a bright smile and welcomed me in. She spoke quickly and confidently, telling me about the errands she needed to do that day, which included taking one of her small dogs to the vet. After the vet, we would go to lunch. Could we take my car?

She didn't mention Bob, the funeral, or GDNF during our trip to the vet. She talked about her dogs and about her work as an interior designer. The visit to the vet went smoothly, and Sherry gave me directions to an Italian restaurant called Bella Vita at the marina, which overlooks the Great Reservoir that wraps around Fishers. When we sat at a small table with a good view of the lake, Sherry Cameron chatted cheerfully about the place and gave me advice on what to order. Her hair was straight and blond and pulled into a bun. She was youthful and pretty. We ordered, and when the waitress left, Sherry looked around and said, "This was one of Bob's favorite places." Her expression grew somber. "We came here all the time."

Sherry met Bob at a community art exhibition when both were well into middle age. Bob was separated from his wife and Sherry was divorced. When Sherry first saw him, she thought Bob looked a lot like the actor William Holden. He was tall, and he had a great smile and a powerful, resonating voice. Marital problems had Bob feeling very discouraged, and the construction supply company he owned was tens of thousands of dollars in debt. He and Sherry began to date in 1991, and the companionship seemed to breathe new life into Bob and restore him to his affable, optimistic self. His company began to flourish.

Bob and Sherry dated during the next five years and were married in 1996. Bob was, Sherry said, the man of her dreams. As a boy, he was an Eagle Scout. In college, he played basketball at Indiana University and was "excessively popular" there and throughout his life. Sherry described Bob as a gifted salesman: "There are the salesmen who are down your throat, those who never give up and don't know when to stop. But Bob did it through some sort of charisma. People knew his word was his bond, and people just trusted him." His company, Triden Construction Supply, employed about 140 people, and it enjoyed steady growth during the couple's first years of marriage.

Bob was diagnosed with Parkinson's disease after the couple had been married only two years. The left side of his body began to deaden and weaken, and his handwriting started to deteriorate. The health of his company mirrored his own, and as Parkinson's took its toll, the company began to falter. In 2003, Bob was forced to take an early retirement that he never would have chosen. Parkinson's forced him to give up golf, which Sherry said was as painful for Bob as any other aspect of the disease. The couple owned a home that overlooked a beautifully manicured golf course, and Bob was desperate to find a way to get back on the course and enjoy the retirement he had anticipated for decades. He became frustrated and despondent. Sherry once calculated that he was taking 6,000 pills per year, but there was no treatment, at any price, that could reverse his condition.

After the meal, we finished our conversation at Sherry's house. The interior was beautifully arranged inside with original artwork on the walls and luxurious furniture. In one wall of the living room was a large, sliding-glass door that opened to the fairway of the golf course just a few steps away. I could imagine how being incapacitated in that place would be maddening to a golf lover.

Sherry sat facing me on one of the couches, and she described Bob's experience on GDNF. He received at most two doses of the drug, but Sherry said she did notice some improvements even in that short window of time. "Bob could smile again, and he had a wonderful smile. He was able to animate his eyes. His face, instead of being frozen, was like he was before. He was able to walk better. He actually was able to get up out of the chair with his own energy. . . . It was like there was this brief moment of hope."

After the trial was halted and it became clear that Amgen wasn't going to reconsider, Bob decided that his condition was too severe to wait. He asked Dr. Penn to remove his pumps and catheters and to replace them with Deep Brain Stimulation, as Amgen had urged. Sherry said DBS did nothing for him, and Bob's decline was swift.

"In January of 2005, he needed a cane, and by March we were really pushing for him to get a walker, which he fought. By June, we were really pushing for him to get a wheelchair, which he also fought. By July, he had a wheelchair and he kind of needed it, and by August, he needed only the wheelchair, and nothing else would work. By Christmas, he really needed a wheelchair, and by February, he couldn't lift himself. He needed help to get out of the bed. And he was total dead weight by March."

The spring weather of 2006 seemed to lift Bob's spirits, and he started to venture out more, which is to say that he allowed Sherry or a caregiver to push him around in a wheelchair. In a happier time, Bob had loved to vacation to Las Vegas, so Sherry planned a trip and talked Bob into going, again with the aid of a caregiver. Bob enjoyed himself so much that he and Sherry planned another trip. This time, it was a road trip to Makinac Island in northern Michigan. The weather was cold and too severe to travel to the island itself, but they went to a small casino at a nearby reservation, where Sherry said Bob enjoyed the same luck that had accompanied him most of his life. "Bob won on the [slot machines]. He always won. The slots always loved him. We were there 15 or 20 minutes and he won $3,000."

Bob seemed content but exhausted as they drove back to Indianapolis. In the days after the trip, he began to cough and wheeze a little, but it seemed like a minor cold that would pass. But his breathing became more labored, and less than three weeks after the road trip, he was hospitalized. Sherry wept openly as she described Bob's final hours in the hospital:

> I went over and put down the rail by the one side of the bed, and I started holding his hand and whispering in his ear and talking to him, and his hand started moving under the cover, and I said, "His hand's moving! His hand's moving!" And so I grabbed his hand under the cover and he held my hand real tight. His daughter came to the other side, and his vitals started to get much worse, much more erratic. So I started talking to him and, I'm not religious, but I didn't want him to die alone. So I started saying things like, "Bob,

you've suffered enough, and God wants to take you now with him because you're a wonderful leader and there are so many problems in the world, and God needs you, and he's preparing you with this horrible illness to go to him and help him. And if you have a chance, you need to go to him, and the Angel's are going to come for you." And his vitals are getting worse, and he's starting to breathe funny. And I'm talking to him saying, "It's okay, honey." And his daughter's saying, "It's okay, Dad. You can go. Don't fight it. It's okay to go." And he held my hand . . . and I said, "Go to the light. Go to God, and it's going to be so wonderful there for you. And I'll see you up there."

And then he breathed a big gasp and kept breathing, and I kept repeating the same things, and then he took one more big gasp and never breathed back out, and he was gone.

41 Richard Hembrough: Twenty-three months after losing GDNF

I flew to England directly from Chicago. I landed at London's Heathrow Airport and took a train two hours to the west toward Bristol. With nearly half a million inhabitants, Bristol is England's sixth-largest city. It received its royal charter in 1155, and every house, wall, barn, and pub seems to be steeped in a history that goes back a dozen generations. The Port of Bristol once was the lifeblood of the local economy and still is identified as the city's cultural center. More recently the aerospace and information technology industries, the film industry, and about nine million tourists a year have outpaced the port as the region's economic engine.

Bristol is one of England's warmest and sunniest cities, and the sun was shining when I stepped off the train at Temple Meads railway station on a late July afternoon. I had arranged to spend several days in the home of Richard Hembrough, the retired middle school teacher. Richard and Patricia still live alongside the rebuilt clock tower in the township of Keynsham. On the top floor of their four-story town home are two small flats that the Hembroughs rent out. One was occupied by a middle-aged man on disability. The other was recently remodeled and vacant, and Richard and Patricia said it would be no trouble to have me stay there during my time in Bristol. Richard surprised me by offering to pick me up from the train station. I was surprised because at the time of our conversation I didn't know exactly when I would be arriving in Bristol, and I assumed he would only be able to drive during his "on" times. He didn't seem concerned, so I thanked him and accepted his offer.

Richard now stood in the station's lobby, leaning his right shoulder against a concrete wall. He is about five-foot-nine with white curly hair and blue eyes that are always open wide, giving him a look of perpetual interest or surprise. When he saw me, he stepped forward to offer his hand in greeting. His movements were stiff but not so odd as to make people stare. He placed each step deliberately and tilted forward slightly as he walked toward me. Richard's voice was soft when he offered a "Hello," and during the drive to his home he spoke relatively little. It wasn't clear whether this was due to shyness or Parkinson's.

Richard and Patricia live about 20 minutes' drive from downtown Bristol, and Richard navigated Bristol's narrow, labyrinthine streets expertly. Their town home is elegant and stately. The limestone is gray and worn, and ivy chases up its outer walls. Inside, the home was undergoing a decade-long remodeling project that began when the Hembroughs moved into the home. There is a large sitting room on the first floor with a fireplace, and one wall is crammed with books and magazines on shelves. When Patricia returned from work at the end of the day, and after dinner at a pub that's within walking distance of their home, she joined me and Richard in the sitting room for an interview.

Patricia Hembrough was in her late fifties with straight auburn hair down to her shoulders. Unlike Stephen, who was shy and soft-spoken, Patricia was warm and garrulous. She still worked as a dentist and was planning to retire very soon. She said she would finally have time to finish remodeling the interior of their home, and she would spend more time tending the garden that wraps around the town house. Like Linda Thacker, Maggie Kaufman, Elaine Suthers, and the other women I met during my travel, Patricia is a devoted caregiver; prior to the trials her life had been as tangled up in the disease as Stephen's. "He was really able to do very little," Patricia said. "He was beginning to get longer and longer times when the medication didn't have any effect. He was starting to become very limited, really."

Whatever Richard couldn't do, Patricia would do for him, all while raising their four children and working full time. Richard got so bad that he was practically immobile during his "off" times, which had grown longer and occurred more frequently. Patricia said that as part of the preparation for the GDNF trial, Richard had to have a PET scan done at Hammersmith Hospital in London, and he had to be completely off of his other medications when he had it done.

"He had to be off his medication overnight," Patricia said, "which was kind of a horrifying thought at the time. And they sent transport for us; they sent a taxi. But he couldn't do anything. In the morning, with no medication overnight, he was really static and needed help to do just about everything." Stephen was nodding with a somber expression.

It occurred to me how unusual it was to be speaking of the ravages of Parkinson's disease in the past tense. Parkinson's doesn't change course or go into remission. It is relentless and unyielding and progressive. No drug on the market can even slow it down. Yet five years after Richard's trip to Hammersmith Hospital in London for the PET scan, he was meeting me at the train station and driving home. He had quit taking his dopamine replacement, Sinemet, about two years into the trial, and though some of his symptoms were slowly reemerging, he hadn't started to take the drugs again. *He was completely off of his medication.*

Patricia must have been thinking the same thing because she said, "When you consider that it's five years on, you would have expected the disease to have moved on, not for him to have improved. But five years on, he's not now taking any of the medication—any of the dopamine. And he's still able to do pretty well, most things. There are times when you wouldn't realize anything's wrong with him now. But more and more before the GDNF it was certainly not the case.

"The improvement, when I think about it—when I think back five years—it's miraculous, really."

42 Stephen Waite: Twenty-three months after losing GDNF

At first, Stephen Waite was not at all interested in talking to me. I had heard from several of his friends that he was very low, very discouraged about how things had transpired after the trial. It was Stephen who had triumphantly returned his disability checks after one year on GDNF. He had traveled with his wife Margaret to Rome at the behest of Amgen to testify of the drug's virtues. And a few months later, he was informed that he would no longer have access to the drug that he credits for changing his life. He did not return my e-mails or my phone calls. In fact, prior to arriving in Bristol, I had never communicated with him directly. I hoped that my coming to Bristol would convince Stephen that I was serious about telling his story.

With Richard Hembrough's help, I finally reached him by phone and asked if he would meet with me and Richard. Stephen reluctantly agreed, and he asked that we meet at the White Harte pub in a small nearby town called Cold Ashton. There was some significance to the spot. It was a place where Stephen had lunch with Richard Hembrough and another patient, Roger Nelson, while the three men were part of the groundbreaking Bristol trial. They met several times during the three years to share a pint and to brag good-naturedly about their improvements ('I drove into town today,' 'I didn't take my pills at all this week,' and so on).

Richard remembers that Stephen was never without a joke, and he always told it with a mischievous twinkle in his eye. The man had a wonderful sense of humor and kept Richard and Roger chuckling throughout the meal. Yet Stephen also seemed to be in a rush all the time, Richard said; he always had a lot of work to do, and, after sharing a drink and a laugh with his mates, he would hurry back to the office.

During an interview with Stephen, his wife Margaret, and Richard in the pub's courtyard, Stephen recalled the months after losing GDNF. He said Amgen stopped the trials at the worst possible time for him. He had just accepted several large and demanding drafting projects, but as the months passed without GDNF, he realized with horror that his hands were growing unsteady. It became harder for him to drive to visit job sites, and it took him considerably longer to finish the projects. Clients grew impatient, projects fell through, and the business floundered.

"We put our house up for sale. We boarded up our little business, sold our house, sold our car. I just made a decision to sell it and that was it."

As disillusioned as he was with Amgen and GDNF, Stephen acknowledged that he continued to benefit from the drug. I asked him a question similar to those I had asked other patients. "Before GDNF, how would this day have been different?"

He looked around and then down at his legs.

"My legs just wouldn't keep still. Prior to the surgery, this table would be turned over right now. My legs would be thrashing about so much. I would've kicked all these glasses over," he said, motioning to our glasses. "That is something that I've kept from GDNF. The bottom half of my body, the legs, have behaved themselves."

Two years after losing GDNF, his legs were noticeably steadier. Five years after his first dose of the drug, his lower half was substantially improved. It was probably little comfort to Stephen, who now walked with a cane, and instead of driving his Jaguar, rode as passenger in his wife's small van. But for a patient with Parkinson's, such improvements were unheard of.

During my interviews with the patients, I often would ask them whether they would do it over again if they had the chance. In each case the patients said that yes, they would do it over again. As painful and exasperating as it was to lose GDNF, the improvements they felt while on the drug justified, in their mind, the agony of losing it.

Stephen Waite was the exception. He surprised me when he said that no, he would not do it again.

"I wouldn't," he said. "I don't think it would be worth it. The last two years or so since this drug was taken away have been the worst of my life. I was just getting the fight back in me again, and it took me 20 years to get that resolved. [GDNF] gave me a false sense of security. I'm finding it very difficult to get that fight back now. It's as if you're not achieving anything in life. You're sitting back and letting people do things for you. It's quite terrible."

43 Dr. Gill

Steve Gill was a complex and rather mysterious figure in the GDNF story. He was the surgeon-inventor who first used a pump to deliver GDNF into the brains of five men in Bristol—and achieved stunning results. On the strength of his results, Amgen sponsored the phase I trial in Kentucky and the multi-center phase II trial. His patients had received GDNF longer than anyone else before Amgen stopped the trials, and they had seen the most striking improvements. The results Dr. Gill achieved in Bristol were the most dramatic of any GDNF clinical trial.

One might expect that Dr. Gill would be the most vocal of the investigators in protesting Amgen's decision, but in fact Dr. Gill was quite reserved in his objections. The e-mails he sent in the days after Amgen halted the trials show his frustration and desperation at the news. But unlike Dr. Hutchinson at NYU, Dr. Slevin and the others at Kentucky, and Dr. Penn in Chicago, Dr. Gill did not offer testimony in support of the patients or for Amgen during the two lawsuits. Nor was he very publicly critical of Amgen, as the others were. His name appeared with the names of Drs. Lang, Nutt, Stacy, and Wooten on the study of the phase II trial—the study that Dr. Hutchinson and the Kentucky doctors refused to co-author because of its conclusions. (Dr. Penn later told me that he had tried to have his name removed from the study but was unable to do so before it was published.) While the other seven principal investigators could easily be categorized as supporting or opposing Amgen's decision, Dr. Gill's position was less clear. It was one of the many things I hoped to find out during our interview.

Like Stephen Waite, Dr. Gill was reluctant to communicate with me at first. I sent half a dozen e-mails and made several phone calls to Frenchay Hospital, all of which went unanswered. Not until I made plans to travel to Bristol did Dr. Gill agree, via his assistant, to meet with me. Of the eight lead investigators, Dr. Gill was the one that I was most anxious to meet. He had pioneered the first successful GDNF trial, and no history of GDNF would be complete without his perspective. After having come so far to search him out, when I finally met him in the waiting room of Frenchay's surgical ward, I said, "Dr. Gill, I presume?"

Physically, Dr. Gill resembles one who might play a neurosurgeon in a movie or television drama. He is about 6 feet tall with a trim, athletic build, a square jaw, and auburn hair. He wears square-frame glasses and is affable, eloquent, and unassuming. I followed him down the ward's narrow, poorly lit corridors to his office. My first thought upon entering was that he had just moved in or else he was preparing to move out. The small boxy room was empty except for a desk, a chair, a computer and some filing cabinets. There was no clutter of any kind. There also was no air conditioning, but Dr. Gill, with his top button undone and his tie loosened a bit, didn't seem to mind.

Dr. Gill had had nearly two years to mull over why the phase II study might have failed and to speculate about Amgen's reasons for stopping the trials. I knew he had a lot to say, but because he had been so reluctant to meet with me at all, I wasn't sure that he would say any of it.

Dr. Gill surprised me by being very open and straightforward during the interview. He said he believed Amgen made a mistake in halting the trials, but he had not been very public in his criticisms because he didn't want to burn bridges with the company. He had seen GDNF work. He was absolutely convinced that it worked. He also knew that Amgen controlled it, at least until the patent expired in 2017, and pitting himself against the company would probably ensure that he would never get GDNF for research purposes again.

So, as difficult as it was, Dr. Gill had kept himself relatively aloof from the debate. Unlike the investigators from Chicago, Kentucky, and New York, he didn't furnish a statement for the patients' lawsuits, nor was he as critical of Amgen in the press. He was conflicted; he wanted to see GDNF returned to his patients, but he needed to stay on good terms with the company that controlled the drug. Perhaps now enough time had passed that he felt he could speak openly about how Amgen's trials fell short.

Dr. Gill had overseen the original Bristol trial that involved five patients. At regular intervals during the trial, he had taken MRI scans of the patients' brains. In addition, Dr. Gill was also one of the seven lead investigators in Amgen's phase II study, for which he had enrolled 10 new patients, each of whom was fitted with the larger catheter, according to Amgen's protocol. Dr. Gill therefore had a unique perspective among the investigators. Five of the patients under his care were receiving GDNF through the catheter he designed, and 10 were receiving the drug through the larger Medtronic catheter that Amgen had chosen.

Because Amgen was not the sponsor of the original GDNF trial in Bristol, Dr. Gill had more autonomy than the investigators of the other two Amgen-sponsored trials. After Amgen halted the trials in September of 2004, Dr. Gill continued to give periodic motor tests to his patients. He wanted to test in as scientific a way as possible how well the patients' improvements were sustained after GDNF was withdrawn. Henry Webb, the first of the five patients, died in December of 2004, before the first follow-up assessment. The other four were assessed six months after losing GDNF, and one patient, Richard Hembrough, was assessed again at one year.

On a timed, left-hand motor test, all four patients scored as well as or better than they had done six months earlier. Three of the four patients were given a complete Unified Parkinson's Disease Rating Scale (UPDRS) assessment six months after losing GDNF. The patients' average off-medication motor score actually improved slightly after six months off of GDNF.

Four years after their first dose of GDNF, the patients' average motor score were improved by 50 percent. That number should be considered in the context of a disease that is supposed to be progressively debilitating. After four and a half years, the patients should have grown worse.

The data was taken from only four patients, making it far from conclusive, but Dr. Gill's had in essence quantified the phenomenon that I had observed informally as I visited the GDNF patients: they were still significantly better off than before GDNF was injected into their lives.

By the time I left Dr. Gill's office, I was convinced that GDNF was the sort of "disease-modifying" drug I had heard Peter Lansbury speak of in Washington D.C. The evidence of sustained improvement had piled so high that attempts to explain it in terms of the placebo effect had become futile.

Total Unified Parkinson's Disease Rating Scale Score for Phase I GDNF Patients in Bristol

This graph shows the results of the UPDRS evaluations for the five Bristol patients, up until the time the trials were halted and the pumps were switched off. Four of the patients were assessed at six months after switch-off, and one patient (Patient 4) was assessed again at one year post switch-off.

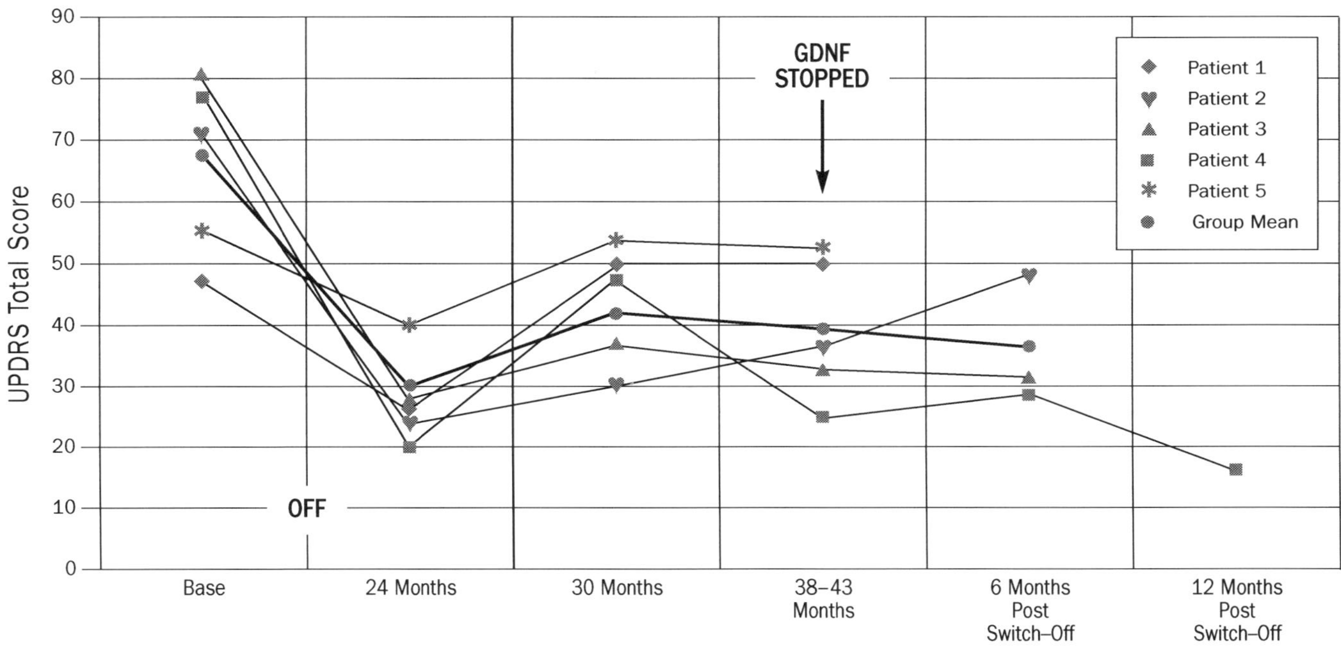

UPDRS Motor Score Assessment for Phase I GNDF Patients in Bristol

This graph shows the results of a UPDRS motor score assessment for the five Bristol patients until the time the trials were halted and the pumps were switched off. Four of the patients were assessed at six months after switch-off, and one patient (Patient 4) was assessed again at one year post switch-off.

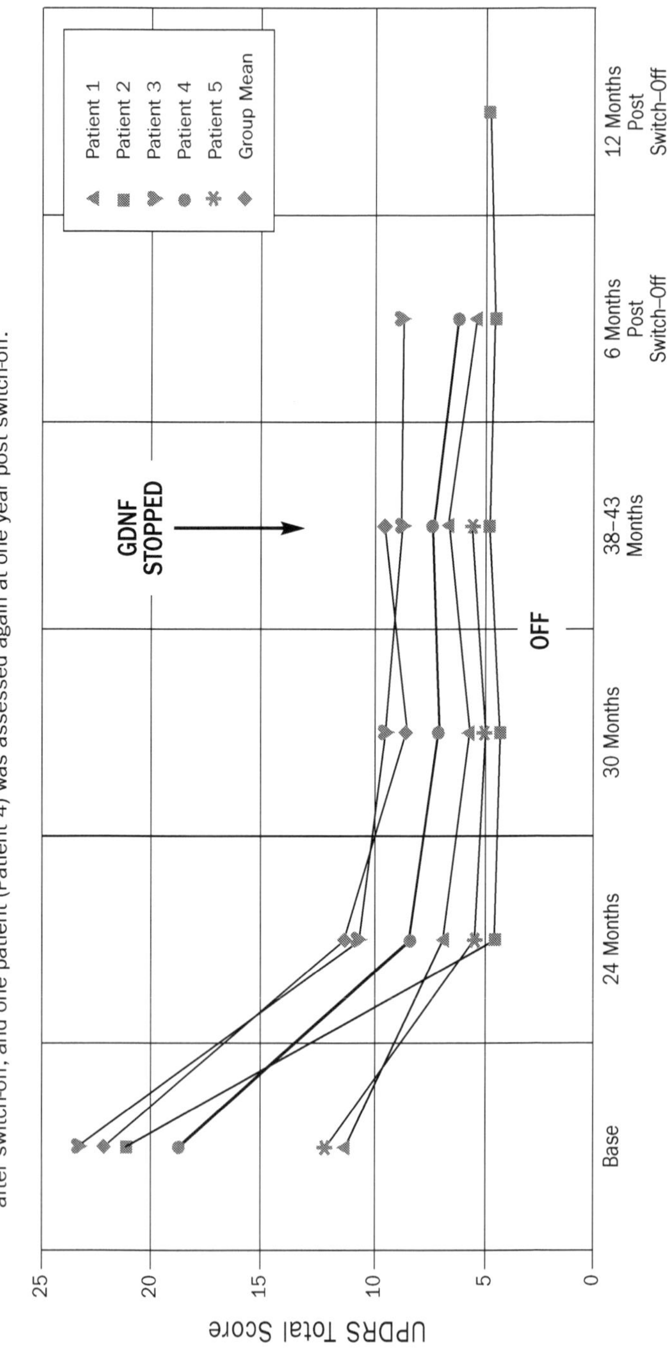

44 Abrupt Withdrawal Revisited

I said goodbye to the Hembroughs and took the train back to London. After my interview with Dr. Gill, I had plenty to think about. I believed that I had found an answer to one of my two largest questions: Does GDNF work? The other question, the one that stilled nagged me as I watched Bristol slip away outside the train window, was 'Is GDNF safe?'

Amgen had said that the pump-and-catheter delivery of GDNF was too risky. First, there were the neutralizing antibodies that had surfaced in a few patients, and second, there was the brain damage, which had been found in four of the 59 monkeys.

By that time, I had heard from several sources inside and outside of Amgen that the antibodies were never a major concern and that, on their own, they would not have been sufficient cause for stopping the trials. Nearly two years after the trials ended, no patient had reported any problems related to the antibodies, and some of the patients who once tested positive for antibodies were now testing negative. In addition, I would later learn that most of the patients found to have antibodies also had had some sort of complication with the pump and catheter. In Bristol, for example, one of the five original patients was found to have antibodies. When that same patient later had his pumps removed, Dr. Gill discovered that the tube that connected the pump to the catheter had become disconnected at the pump end. For an unknown period, which might have been more than three years, the GDNF was pumped directly into the patient's abdomen. He was the only patient in Bristol to test positive for antibodies. There were similar cases in Toronto and Kentucky, where the patients who developed antibodies were also the patients who had some device-related issues.

During a conference call with several lead investigators in February of 2005, Amgen's head of research and development, Roger Perlmutter, said his concerns about the brain damage eclipsed any concerns about the antibodies.

"I'm much less concerned about the antibody question," he said. "I'm *really* concerned about cerebellar toxicity."

The brain damage in the four monkeys had always been, and continued to be, the most troubling issue. One of the recommendations that came out of the GDNF summit that the Michael J. Fox Foundation organized in October 2004 was that the primate toxicology study should be repeated. Amgen had not followed the advice, nor had any of the research institutions repeated the expensive study.

Dr. Hutchinson and others continued to argue that the *abrupt withdrawal* of GDNF had caused the brain damage. Three of the four monkeys had received high doses of the drug for six months and then had it abruptly taken away. The existence of that fourth monkey, however, the one that supposedly received GDNF right up until the time of its death, seriously undermined the withdrawal phenomenon explanation.

Or did it?

I spoke with several sources who were close to the trials and who had seen Amgen's data from the toxicology study. After several phone interviews and on condition of anonymity, three sources independently told me that Amgen was not revealing all of the important data. They said the fourth monkey did indeed have GDNF pumped into its brain at a very high dose until the time of its death. But they said there was more to the story, and Amgen wasn't telling it.

As part of the toxicology study, Amgen tested the monkeys' cerebosprinal fluid at two points: once at the beginning of the study, shortly after the pumps were turned on, and once again at six months, just before the monkeys were sacrificed. The tests were to determine whether there was any GDNF mixed in with the cerebrospinal fluid. If there was, that meant the GDNF was probably being delivered properly to the brain. If not, it meant GDNF wasn't getting into the brain as it should. It meant that there had been some kind of interruption.

According to the three sources who said they had seen the data, the fourth monkey was tested at the commencement of the study and showed the expected levels of GDNF in its fluid. But when the monkey was tested again at six months, just before being sacrificed, the GDNF levels in the fluid had dropped significantly. The drop suggested that at some point between the first month and the six month there had been an interruption, an *abrupt withdrawal* that was not intended.

With this new information, the picture became much clearer. All four of the damaged monkeys had been treated with extremely high doses of GDNF for several months. Three of them were abruptly withdrawn from the drug at six months, according to plan. But this new bit of information suggests that the fourth monkey had also been abruptly withdrawn, and though the withdrawal was not planned, its effect on the brain would have been the same. Perhaps a tube had become kinked or disconnected, or maybe the pump malfunctioned.

When I reviewed the court documents that described the toxicology study, I learned that originally 72 monkeys had been implanted with pumps and catheters for the study. According to the court documents, thirteen of them died or were euthanized because of complications with the pumps and catheters. I asked Amgen to elaborate on what sorts of things occasioned the deaths of the 13 monkeys. Amgen responded with the following:

> Ten animals were euthanized and one animal died because of pump-site-related problems, such as skin erosions due to the relatively large size of the pump in relation to the size of the animal. One animal was euthanized because of an irreversible pump malfunction. In addition, one monkey in the mid-dose group was euthanized with clinical signs and clinical pathology findings consistent with disseminated intravascular coagulation (DIC) during study week 15. Microscopic evaluation of this animal revealed widespread hemorrhages.

In other words, the study was a mess. A full 20 percent of the monkeys that originally were enrolled had died or were euthanized before the study began. Is it a great stretch to suppose that a similar breakdown occurred in that fourth monkey?

The quasi-independent group that Amgen had commissioned in 2004 to analyze the toxicology study had discarded the withdrawal-phenomenon explanation because of the existence of the fourth monkey. The question of withdrawal phenomenon was barely mentioned during the legal hearings for the same reason. Yet this new information about the unintended withdrawal in that fourth monkey makes an even more compelling case for Dr. Hutchinson's withdrawal phenomenon explanation. Of the 15 primates that got the very high dose of GDNF, four had suffered brain damage, and according to the new information, all four had been abruptly withdrawn.

When Amgen officials first learned that brain damage had been discovered in two monkeys, they were understandably alarmed. It was strange, it was unprecedented, and the news of it came just as Amgen was considering an *increase* in the dose in humans. The news also came on the heels of the failed phase II study, which from the company's perspective tipped the risk-benefit evaluation in the direction of stopping the trials. The decision to cancel the trials could affect the performance of Amgen's stock, so only a select number of Amgen scientists would be involved in the discussion, and none of the outside investigators would be. GDNF's champion within Amgen, the respected Mickey Traub, had died months earlier. The man who had gone to the mat for GDNF time and time again was gone, and no one internally had stepped up to replace him in that role.

The group chose to err on the side of caution (medically and legally), and Amgen's leaders ordered the trials stopped. The patients' pumps were to be switched off immediately and removed as soon as possible. In effect, Amgen ordered an abrupt withdrawal. Not until weeks later did Dr. Hutchinson at NYU suggested that withdrawal phenomenon could account for the brain damage, which at that point had been discovered in only two monkeys. Amgen had a clear incentive to reject the withdrawal phenomenon explanation. If suddenly losing the drug had harmed the monkeys, then by withdrawing the drug from the patients, the company would have unintentionally exposed them to the very risk it wished to avoid.

Perhaps that is why Amgen chose not to replicate the toxicology study, as they had been advised to do. Perhaps the company would rather not find out, definitively, whether abrupt withdrawal of GDNF had caused the brain damage.

By the time the summit took place, Amgen was already thick into talks with Martha Bohn at Northwestern University and Howard Federoff at the University of Rochester about delivering GDNF through gene therapy. There would be no bulky metal pumps or plastic tubes threaded under the skin. Gene therapy was looking more promising by the day, while the Medtronic pumps, based on 1970s technology, were looking more and more like a neurosurgical dinosaur.

There was little to be gained financially, from Amgen's perspective, in pursuing a treatment that couldn't be administered to all who needed it. Recall that during his speech to students at the University of California, Davis, Amgen's Roger Perlmutter said the lengthy, complex operation that GDNF requires wasn't feasible on a large scale. "There aren't enough neurosurgeons in the country to do that procedure, and there aren't enough neurosurgical suites in which to do it, so that will limit you pretty dramatically."

The company was ready to move on.

45 Tom Isaacs

Tom Isaacs had invited me to visit him in his home in northern London before I returned to the United States. Tom was the man who had trekked across the entire coastline of Britain in one year to raise money for Parkinson's research. It was Tom who put together the before-and-after video I had seen in Washington D.C., and it was Tom who helped me to contact Dr. Gill and his patients in Bristol. I wanted to thank him in person for his help.

When his medication is working, Tom is a youthful, charismatic man in his late 30s. He has brown curly hair, he's witty and spry, and he's married to a lovely Scottish woman named Lyndsey. Together they have a small dog named Chewbacca. Tom drives a blue convertible sports car and navigates London's Underground rail system with ease. He matched this description for at least 90 percent of the time I spent with him over two days.

For the other 10 percent of the time, Tom would excuse himself and retire to a back room. He would return an hour or so later with his shirt damp from perspiration and with his hair all a mess. I had become used to these interruptions during interviews with other patients. The person would begin to tremble and then would apologize and leave the room. I would wait out the storm that I knew was raging behind the closed doors. Tom's intermittent exits were not unusual. On the second day of my visit, however, Tom did something no patient had done before. He let me watch the disease overtake him.

We had just finished eating lunch when Tom looked at his watch, breathed out a long sigh, and predicted his body's rebellion like a seismologist forecasting a quake. He said he had taken his medication too soon after eating, and the medication wasn't going to kick in before his morning dose wore off. About 30 minutes later, when his fingertips began to tremble, he didn't excuse himself, as he had done before. He took a few wavering steps to the living room, lay on the carpet and said that it was all right, I didn't have to leave. It was upon him within a few minutes.

His head shook furiously and his tongue wagged between his lips. His mouth curled into an unnatural joker's smile. His arms bent at the elbow and pumped in tight jerks while his snarled fingers flailed in front of his chest like the limbs of a frenzied conductor. His torso was rigid, and crimson sweat marks were appearing where his bright red polo shirt pressed against his damp skin. He lay on his side, propped up by an overstuffed beige throw pillow.

Only the pupils of his eyes were still, or they appeared so to me because he kept them fixed on me despite the jerking of his head. He was watching me watch him. He wanted me to see him like this. This was my real education. *This* was Parkinson's disease.

I remembered in that moment the flapping and writhing of the interpretive dancer on the stage in Washington D.C., which at the time had baffled me. The dance had seemed chaotic and overdone. Now I understood it. I also understood why Dave Heydrick reacted as he did when he saw it, why he grew emotional and said, "I hope

I never get to be like that." She, the dancer who lost a father to Parkinson's, and he, the neurologist who treated patients in advanced stages of the disease, had seen many times what I was now seeing in Tom Isaacs's living room. In the preceding months, I had interviewed dozens of Parkinson's patients and some of the world's most accomplished neurologists. I had read books and articles in medical journals on the disease. I had learned much about Parkinson's, and now, finally, I was looking at the disease itself.

Tom never received GDNF. He was not one of those 50 patients who had it pumped into their brains between 2001 and 2004. But he saw the before-and-after videos of Stephen Waite and Richard Hembrough; he read the reports about Roger Thacker, Bob Suthers, and Steve Kaufman in the United States. In Bristol, he met Dr. Gill. Like thousands of other Parkinson's patients, he had watched GDNF as it inched toward him down the drug pipeline—an excruciatingly slow process for a patient with a progressive, degenerative disease. In the fall of 2004 he saw it all fall apart. Amgen halted the trials indefinitely, and, just like that, GDNF was gone. Two years later, around the time GDNF was to have made its debut onto the commercial market, I was watching Tom Isaacs as he lay, shaking, on his living room floor.

AFTERWORD

In the year that has passed between the completion of this manuscript and its publication, Amgen has announced no new testing of GDNF, and the company continues to forbid use of the drug in clinical trials. The attention of the Parkinson's community has shifted to a California-based company called Ceregene Inc. and its product, CERE-120. Ceregene reportedly approached Amgen in 2005 in the hopes of licensing GDNF for gene therapy delivery. After Amgen declined, the company instead used a cousin of GDNF called neurturin for its product CERE-120, which is essentially a virus that has been reengineered to deliver neurturin to the human brain. The Michael J. Fox Foundation helped to fund a phase I test of CERE-120, and the results were comparable to those achieved by Dr. Steven Gill in Bristol. Enrollment for a phase II test was completed in late 2007. According to a Ceregene press release, clinical data from the phase II are expected to be available in late 2008, and if the data are positive, a phase III trial is expected to commence in 2009.

In a development that many Parkinson's patients must attribute to karma, Amgen's stock has suffered of late, arguably as a result of the company's inability to innovate. Two of Amgen's blockbuster drugs, which together make up about 40 percent of the company's revenue, have come under fire. The first is Epogen, Amgen's original blockbuster. For the first time, the drug faces direct competition on U.S. soil from Switzerland-based Roche Holding. Amgen prevailed in a patent infringement suit against Roche, but rather than prohibit Roche from selling its product in the United States, the judge merely required Roche to pay a royalty to Amgen on any sales. As a result, Amgen now must compete in a market it once monopolized.

The other drug, Aranesp, has proven even more problematic. Aranesp is a slightly modified, longer-acting version of Epogen. In early 2007, Amgen revealed that in a trial of 1,000 patients who suffered from anemia as a result of cancer, Aranesp increased the risk of death and did nothing to alleviate the anemia. That study and others prompted the FDA to require "black box" warnings about the risks of Aranesp, and in early 2008 an FDA panel considered removing the drug from the market altogether. The panel stopped short of an outright ban but did recommend severe restrictions on how Aranesp may be prescribed. The result of these complications is that Amgen's stock has tumbled from about $75 per share in early 2007 to less than $40 per share in 2008. Once the undisputed leader in biotech, Amgen now fights for third place with Gilead Sciences Inc., with both of them trailing far behind Genentech in terms of market capitalization. The company's financial woes have given some patients hope that the company may be more willing to sell or license GDNF, but Amgen has said nothing of this so far.

In March of 2007, Bob Suthers began to have greater difficulty moving around the house. By May, he could no longer get out of his chair without help. Concerned that his Parkinson's was advancing quickly, Elaine took him to a doctor, who told her that the new symptoms weren't caused by Parkinson's. Bob was in the advanced stages of mesothilioma, probably brought on by his exposure to asbestos during his career in the textile industry. He died a little more than one week later. Elaine said that even though Bob didn't die of Parkinson's, she still felt that the suddenness of Bob's death was in part because of Amgen's decision to halt the GDNF trials. She said Amgen "took good years away from Bob that he otherwise would have had." He might have continued to improve, but instead, he had spent almost two years fighting the company for access to GDNF, hiring an attorney, scrawling angry letters, fuming at the injustice of the situation. Elaine also said that Bob's relapse after losing GDNF made it more difficult to distinguish the symptoms of the mesothilioma when they emerged. "I keep thinking that if Amgen hadn't taken away the drug, he would have been healthy enough that we would have recognized the symptoms—that it wasn't Parkinson's," she said.

In December of 2007, more than three years after the GDNF trials were halted, Amgen finally published the results of its primate toxicology study.[54] The study confirmed what sources had revealed to me on condition of anonymity—that the samples taken from the fourth monkey suggest that the animal experienced an inadvertent withdrawal of GDNF. According to the study, an initial sample of the cerebrospinal fluid (CSF) was taken from each monkey one month into the study. Another sample was taken at the end of the six-month treatment. Recall that some of the monkeys also underwent a three-month "recovery" period, during which time the monkeys were kept alive but did not receive GDNF. From the monkeys in this group, an additional CSF sample was taken at the end of the recovery period. Of the four monkeys that were found to be brain damaged, three had passed through the three-month recovery period, which suggested that the withdrawal of GDNF at the six-month mark had caused the damage. The fourth monkey, however, had not been through the recovery period. It hadn't been *intentionally* withdrawn from GDNF, which had prompted Amgen's scientists to reject Dr. Michael Hutchinson's withdrawal phenomenon explanation.

The study data show that there were high levels of GDNF in the fluid of the fourth monkey in the initial sample, the sample collected one month into the study. But the sample collected from the same monkey five months later showed *non-detectable* levels of GDNF. This suggests that some interruption occurred during those five months and that the interruption effectively cut off the flow of GDNF to the monkey's brain. According to the study, the small number of monkeys involved and the infrequency of CSF sampling didn't allow for "definitive conclusions" about the possibility of withdrawal phenomenon. However, the study authors did concede that "this possibility warrants further investigation."

After reading an early draft of the manuscript for this book, an acquaintance wrote, "Great work, but I am also interested in what happened to you. What happened at your paper? Did you get another job?" The truth is that I did write to my former managing editor about the possibility of reporting for the paper again. The letter went unreturned. It was all right, though, because by that time I had applied to several law schools, and I knew I wouldn't be in South Texas much longer. I worked briefly as an investigative reporter for KZTV Action 10 News, a CBS affiliate in Corpus Christi, before moving east to study at the University of Virginia School of Law. On the drive from Texas to Virginia, we stopped to visit Roger and Linda Thacker.

It had been a hot August day, but we arrived at the home in the evening when the air had cooled. I maneuvered the moving van up the gravel driveway. During my previous visit, I had been alone.

Now, I was accompanied by my wife, our toddler daughter, and our infant son. As she had done before, Linda emerged from the home as the vehicle rolled to a stop. She greeted us warmly and let us in. Roger was in his bedroom and out of sight (Linda apologized that he was "off" at the moment). The rest of us visited in the living room for a while, and then Linda said that dinner must be ready and asked us to sit around the table. At some point during the meal, Roger became sufficiently "on" or just sufficiently hungry to join us. Linda helped him cross the room to a tall chair. His head rocked back and forth, and the movements of his legs and arms were stiff and unsure. He didn't sit in the chair but rather propped himself against it as Linda helped him to eat.

My wife later told me that when Roger had entered the room, she had felt uneasy and unsure how to act or what to say. It was her first time in the company of a person with advanced Parkinson's. Her words reminded me of my own unease when I attended the annual forum of the Parkinson's Action Network in Washington D.C. in early 2006. That had been my first time. Now, visiting Roger more than a year later, I felt none of the awkwardness of before. My wife's words reminded me of how isolating Parkinson's can be. I thought of Bob Suthers and how he related that friends and relatives had stopped visiting him because they were put off by the look of apathy that the disease plastered upon his face. It was a disease that not only robbed the use of the body and deadened the pleasure centers of the brain but also deprived its sufferers of the very relationships that could make the whole experience bearable.

Roger eventually did come back "on" again, and we chatted for a while about the work he had been doing on the farm and about his future plans for the property. It was during that discussion that I noticed the change in Roger and Linda. They no longer seemed preoccupied with Amgen and the halted trials, which had dominated their thoughts and speech during my previous visit. The maddening frustration at the injustice of it all seemed to have left them. Instead, Roger spoke about Linda's children, how he enjoyed having them close and seeing the grandchildren often. He talked excitedly about a new business venture he was planning, hoping that it would be very profitable. His focus, and hers, was on the future and not the past.

And why not? The couple had stood together in their fight for GDNF for nearly three years. They had written countless letters, had spoken to a dozen reporters, hoping to sway the court of public opinion in their favor. They had pursued a legal remedy by taking Amgen to court. Had they won the day, it would have been a David and Goliath tale for the ages. Yet at some point, the Thackers must have realized that they could spend the rest of their lives battling Amgen for access to GDNF. Their bitterness and contempt for the company could accrue year by year until it consumed every thought. In the end, though, they may have nothing to show for it except a lake of bitterness and a lot of wasted years. One could hardly fault a couple in the twilight of life for deciding to cherish the present and look to the future rather than dwell on an injustice of the past.

Yet Parkinson's remains a part of our future, and the need to cure it also remains. Perhaps it falls upon the rest of us—those who have not yet reached life's twilight—to take up that struggle as our own. As I wrote in this book's preface, I am not a scientist, and I have not set out with this book to prove that GDNF or any other drug is a cure for Parkinson's. Perhaps my part in the struggle toward a cure is simply to recount the experiences of Roger Thacker, Bob Suthers, and the other GDNF patients. I offer their stories, as James Parkinson once wrote, "with the pleasing hope that they may lessen the number of victims to negligence and presumption."

NOTES

1. Steven S. Gill, et al., "Direct Brain Infusion of Glial Cell-Line-Derived Neurotrophic Factor [GDNF] in Parkinson's Disease," *Nature Medicine,* May 2003, p. 589 and *also* Nikunj K. Patel, et al., "Intraputamenal Infusion of [GDNF] in PD: A Two-Year Outcome Study," *Annals of Neurology*, February 2005, p. 298.

2. National Center for Health Statistics, "Deaths: Final Data for 2004," January 2007. Obtainable at http://www.cdc.gov/nchs/products/pubs/pubd/hestats/finaldeaths04/finaldeaths04_tables.pdf#2 and *also* "Deaths: Final Data for 2003" January 2007, at http://www. cdc.gov/nchs/data/hestat/finaldeaths03_tables.pdf.

3. Oliver Sacks, *Awakenings,* Duckworth, London, 1973.

4. The National Parkinson's Foundation, founded in 1957, took in $8.4 million in direct contributions in 2005. The Parkinson's Disease Foundation, also founded in 1957, took in $6.3 million. The American Parkinson's Disease Association, founded in 1961, had $12.9 million in direct contributions. *See* IRS form 990 for each company, obtainable at www.guidestar.org.

5. Academy of Achievement, "Interview: Jonas Salk, M.D.," May 16, 1991. Obtainable at http://www.achievement.org/autodoc/page/sal0int-1.
6. D. Schubert, et al., "Clonal Cell-Lines from the Rat Central Nervous System," *Nature,* May 1974, p. 224.
7. M. Churchill Bohn, and M. Kanuicki, "Bilateral Recovery of Dopamine After Unilateral Adrenal Grafting into the Striatum of the [MPTP]-Treated Mouse," *Journal of Neuroscience Research,* March 1990, p. 281.
8. J. Engele, D. Schubert, and M.C. Bohn, "Conditioned Media Derived from Glial Cell Lines Promote Survival and Differentiation of Dopaminergic Neurons In Vitro: Role of mesencephalic glia," *Journal of Neuroscience Research,* October 1991, p. 359.
9. Leu-Fen Lin, et al., "GDNF: a glial cell line-derived neurotrophic factor for midbrain dopaminergic neurons," *Science,* May 21, 1993, p. 1130.
10. "Septic Shock Claims Another Victim," *Applied Genetics News,* August 1994.
11. Andrew Pollack, "Many See Hope in Parkinson's Drug Pulled from Testing," *New York Times,* November 26, 2004, p. A1.
12. Robert Langreth, "Biotech Behemoth," *Forbes,* January 10, 2005.
13. A. Tomac, "Protection and Repair of the Nigrostriatal Dopaminergic System by GDNF In Vivo," *Nature,* January 26, 1995. *See also* Z. Zhang, "Dose Response to Intraventricular Glial Cell Line-Derived Neurotrophic Factor Administration in Parkinsonian Monkeys," *Journal of Pharmacology and Experimental Therapeutics,* September 1997, p. 1396.

14. J.G. Nutt, et al. "Randomized, Double-Blind Trial of [GDNF] in PD," *Neurology,* January 14, 2003, p. 69. *See also* Jeffrey Kordower, et al., "Clinico-Pathological Findings Following Intraventricular GDNF Treatment in a Patient with Parkinson's Disease," *American Academy of Neurology 51st Annual Meeting,* April 18, 1999.

15. *Ibid.*

16. Elizabeth White, "St. John the Baptist: A history of the church," Malago Press & Print Services, Bristol, 2005, pp. 22–26.

17. "Deep Brain Stimulation," University of Maryland Medical Center Departments of Neurology and Neurosurgery, accessed August 2006. Obtainable at http://www.umm.edu/neurosciences/deep_brain.html

18. Steven S. Gill, et al., "Direct Brain Infusion of Glial Cell-Line-Derived Neurotrophic Factor [GDNF] in Parkinson's Disease," *Nature Medicine,* May 2003, p. 589

19. Nikunj K. Patel, et al., "Intraputamenal Infusion of [GDNF] in PD: A Two-Year Outcome Study," *Annals of Neurology,* February 2005, p. 298.

20. *Ibid.*

21. Pallab Ghosh, "Parkinson's Brain Renewal Advance," BBC Web site, April 18, 2002. Obtainable at http://news.bbc.co.uk/2/hi/science/nature/1935593.stm.

22. John T. Slevin, et al., "Improvement of Bilateral Motor Functions in Patients with Parkinson's Disease Through the Unilateral Intraputaminal Infusion of [GDNF]," *Journal of Neurosurgery*, February 2005, p. 216.

23. Anthony E. Lang, et al., "Randomized Controlled Trial of Intraputamenal [GDNF] in Parkinson's Disease," *Annals of*

Neurology, December 2005, p. 459.

24. *Ibid.*

25. A 2003 study of rats found that DDT was especially damaging to the dopamine-producing cells affected by Parkinson's disease. The study concluded that "exposure to DDT from contaminated environments is therefore a potential risk of onset of Parkinson's disease." *See* K.W. Leung, et al. "[DDT] Specifically Depletes Dopaminergic Neurons in Primary Cell Culture," *Neuroembryology,* 2003, p. 95.

26. Video of full Roger Perlmutter's keynote address is accessible online at: http://www.uctv.tv/library-test.asp?showID=8901

27. *Ibid.*

28. Anthony E. Lang, et al., "Randomized Controlled Trial of Intraputamenal [GDNF] Infusion in Parkinson's Disease," *Annals of Neurology,* December 2005, p. 459.

29. "Amgen's Phase 2 Study of GDNF for Advanced Parkinson's Disease Fails to Meet Primary Endpoint; Six Months of Treatment Showed Biological Effect But No Clinical Improvement." Press release accessible online at http://www-ext.amgen.com/media/media_pr_detail.jsp?year=2004&releaseID= 585632

30. "Affidavit of Mark T. Butt, D.V.M.," *Suthers v. Amgen Inc.,* United States District Court, Southern District of New York, Case No. 05-cv-4158.

31. "Affidavit of Roger M. Perlmutter, M.D., Ph.D.," *Suthers v. Amgen Inc.,* United States District Court, Southern District of New York, Case No. 05-cv-4158.

32. "Affidavit of Mark T. Butt, D.V.M.," *Suthers v. Amgen Inc.,* United States Court of Appeals for the Second Circuit, Docket No. 05-254.

33. Todd B. Sherer, "Crossroads in GDNF Therapy for Parkinson's Disease," *Movement Disorders,* February 2006, p. 136.

34. *Ibid.*

35. *Ibid.*

36. *Ibid.*

37. *Ibid.*

38. *Ibid.*

39. M.L. Florez-McClure, et al., "The p75 Neurotrophin Receptor Can Induce Autophagy and Death of Cerebellar Purkinje Neurons," *Journal of Neuroscience,* May 12, 2004, p. 4498.

40. Sherer, Todd B., "Crossroads in GDNF Therapy for Parkinson's Disease," *Movement Disorders,* February 2006, p. 136.

41. Ms. Martin's and all other quotations from this chapter are taken from court filings associated with *Suthers v. Amgen Inc.*, United States District Court, Southern District of New York, Case No. 05-cv-4158.

42. All quotations from this chapter are taken from the certified transcript of the preliminary hearing for *Suthers v. Amgen Inc.*, United States District Court, Southern District of New York, Case No. 05-cv-4158.

43. All quotations from this chapter are taken from the certified transcript of the preliminary hearing for *Abney v. Amgen Inc.*, United States District Court, Eastern District of Kentucky, case No. 5:05-cv-00254-JMH.

44. S. Love, et al., "[GDNF] Induces Neuronal Sprouting in Human Brain," *Nature Medicine,* July 2005, p. 703.

45. *Ibid.*

46. Excerpts from the *60 Minutes* report are accessible online at http://www.cbsnews.com/stories/2005/09/08/60minutes/main828098.shtml

47. Anthony E. Lang, et al., "GDNF Treatment of Parkinson's Disease: Response to editorial," *Lancet Neurology,* March 2006, p. 200.

48. R.D. Penn, et al., "GDNF Treatment of Parkinson's Disease: Response to editorial," *Lancet Neurology,* March 2006, p. 202.

49. R.A. Barker, "Continuing Trials of GDNF in Parkinson's Disease," *Lancet Neurology,* April 2006, p. 285.

50. Anthony E. Lang, et al., "Randomized Controlled Trial of Intraputamenal [GDNF] Infusion in Parkinson's Disease," *Annals of Neurology,* December 2005, p. 459.

51. M. Hutchinson, "GDNF in Parkinson's Disease: An object lesson in the tyranny of type II," *Journal of Neuroscience Methods,* July 27, 2006.

52. Andrew Pollack, "Many See Hope in Parkinson's Drug Pulled from Testing," *New York Times,* November 26, 2004, p. A1.

53. Paula Moyer, "GDNF Showed No Benefit in Parkinson's Disease Trial; Study Discontinued," *Neurology Today,* November 2004.

54. D. Hovland, et al., "Six-Month Continuous Intraputamenal Infusion Toxicity Study of Recombinant Methionyl Human Glial Gell Line-Derived Neurotrophic Factor (r-metHuGDNF) in Rhesus Monkeys," *Toxicology Pathology,* December 2007, p. 1013.

INDEX

ABOUT THE AUTHOR

Nick Nelson received his BA in Journalism from Brigham Young University. He reported for the *Daily Herald* in Provo, Utah and then at the *Corpus Christi Caller-Times* in South Texas, where he won awards from the Dallas Press Association and the Texas Associated Press Managing Editors Association. After completing the manuscript for *Monkeys in the Middle,* Nick worked briefly as an investigative reporter for KZTV Action 10 News in Corpus Christi before commencing his studies at the University of Virginia School of Law. Nick, his wife Nadine, and their two children live in Charlottesville, Virginia.

Made in the USA
Lexington, KY
09 August 2012